I0114870

Praise for *I AM Intuitive*

The journey inward is reflected in all aspects of your life. It takes courage to meet yourself. Dr. Dijamco deeply understands these concepts—the inner workings of what makes us human—and weaves simple practices that you can incorporate into your own life journey. She has a warmth and compassion that's been evident since meeting her years ago at Dr. Andrew Weil's Integrative Medicine Fellowship at the University of Arizona. *I AM Intuitive* is for truth-seekers, empaths and anyone with the desire to know themselves.

> — TIERAONA LOW DOG, MD
> author of National Geographic's *Life is Your Best Medicine*

I am recommending Dr. Arlene Dijamco's book, *I AM Intuitive*, to my loved ones. It is a book I wish I had written. She introduces many practical exercises for achieving the highest level of health by addressing the whole human being – body, mind, and spirit. Congratulations to Arlene for creating a blueprint for proactive self-care and for finally and fearlessly birthing, against staid habits and beliefs of conventional medicine, a truly effective template for all of healthcare!

> — PAUL LEE, DO, FAAO, FCA, DABMA
> author of *Interface: Mechanisms of Spirit in Osteopathy*

I trained Dr. Dijamco to practice Reiki during her medical residency, as she was exploring the interface of medicine and spirituality, and developing a more expansive understanding of health and healing. I was impressed by her equanimity, her inquiring mind, and her open heart. I'm so pleased she's bringing what she's learned works well for her patients to a wider public.

> — PAMELA MILES, internationally-renowned Reiki Master, foremost Medical Reiki expert, author of the award-winning book *REIKI: A Comprehensive Guide*

We are pleased to recommend *I AM Intuitive* by Dr. Arlene Dijamco. This book will encourage you to explore, your mind, body, and spirit, while guiding you to find a clear path for your search of freedom and purpose within your own life. An incredible reference book to empower you with inspiring feelings, thoughts, words, and actions.

> — MAUDY FOWLER AND GAIL HUNT, international award-winning authors of *Angel Whispers: Messages of Hope and Healing from Loved Ones*

I cannot wait to get this book into the hands of everyone I know! Arlene's gift of fearlessly weaving together science and spirit is on full display in this beautiful, highly practical manual for everyone interested in living into every dimension of what it means to be human.

> — CORINNE CAYCE, integral leadership coach

I AM
intuitive

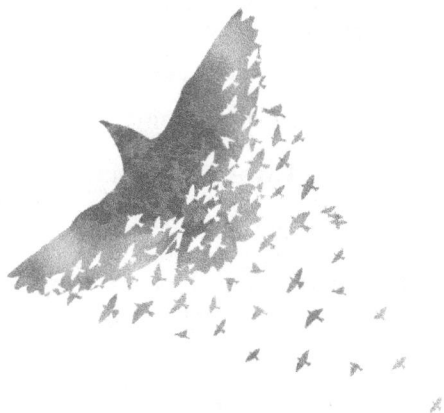

I AM
intuitive

A MultiDimensional Guide
to Embrace Your Inner Light

Arlene Dijamco, MD, FAAP

all worlds
-PRESS-

all worlds
-PRESS-

Roswell, GA
allworldspress.com

Copyright © 2024 by Arlene Dijamco, MD

All rights reserved.

No part of this book may be reproduced or used in any manner without written permission of the copyright owner except for the use of quotations in a book review.

First edition 2024

Book design by Diane Rigoli - RigoliCreative.com

ISBN: 978-1-963899-01-6 (paperback)
978-1-963899-00-9 (hardcover)
978-1-963899-06-1 (audiobook)
978-1-963899-04-7 (e-book)

LCCN: 2024913452

DISCLAIMER:
The information in this book is for informational purposes only. The information in this book is the author's opinion and is not intended as a substitute for the advice provided by your physician or other healthcare professional. You should not use the information in this book for diagnosing or treating a health problem or disease, or for prescribing any medication or other treatment. Buying or reading this book does not form a physician-patient relationship with Dr. Arlene Dijamco. Consult with a healthcare professional directly before implementing any changes to your health regimen, and do not delay seeking treatment because of something you have read in this book.

Please note: this book addresses stress, trauma, and other challenging life experiences with gentleness, kindness, love, honor, and respect. If you have had severe trauma, please work directly with a qualified trauma medical or mental-health professional.

Although the stories in this book are real, most names and identifying details have been changed to protect the privacy of certain individuals.

To Dad, in spirit

Who am I?
> *You are love,* said the Stillness
> *A unique emanation of the Divine.*

Why do I see shadows?
> *They are but an illusion*
> *An eclipsing of the heart.*

Where is my light?
> *Shining always within you*
> *For you are a living rainbow*
> *Love in motion.*

Remember who you are.

CONTENTS

Preface

Hi. My name is Arlene Dijamco. I'm an integrative physician, a pediatrician, and a cranial osteopath. I've studied at Harvard University, Emory University, and Albert Einstein College of Medicine, as well as Dr. Andrew Weil's Center for Integrative Medicine, where I did a fellowship in integrative medicine. While my formal education gave me a solid background in science and medicine, that hasn't ended my education—I am a forever student. I attribute much of my education to my interactions with patients and my life experiences. Through it all, I've learned to value and trust my intuition.

My mission is to help bring the intuitive spirit back to medicine in practical and tangible ways. We don't have to try to get in touch with Spirit because *we are spiritual beings*. It's our nature—so there's an ease to aligning mind, body, and spirit. I hope reading this book will help you step into the ease of intuitive living.

INTRODUCTION

When I was in medical school, I met a woman hospitalized with pneumonia at Grady, Atlanta's public hospital. I'll call this woman Doris. I was on rounds with the other med students. We were learning how to interview patients and record detailed histories—something we wouldn't have time to do once we were physicians (or so we were told). I asked Doris every question on my list, from the mundane to the intimate, like this one:

"Have you ever been sexually abused?"

"Yes," said Doris.

My eyebrows rose. I looked at the next question.

"Have you ever told anyone?" I asked.

"No."

I looked at my paper. There were no follow-up questions given for that answer. Doris had just revealed a traumatic event in her life for the first time ever—to a wide-eyed group of medical students. And no one said a peep, not even the attending physician.

I wanted to cry, for myself and Doris.

At that time in my life, I couldn't always tell whose emotions I was feeling because they felt all mixed up. Were they my emotions or someone else's? At that moment, did it matter? Because either way, I knew what was happening was unfair. As physicians in training, who had made a Hippocratic oath to "first do no harm," we were obligated to help Doris. If we didn't acknowledge or address her traumatic event as if she was a person who mattered, then we were doing a great disservice. She deserved to be treated as a whole human being, not just a physical body.

I wanted to scream.

The next day, we had an ethics group meeting to discuss delicate matters like this. I shared the story of what Doris had said, how she had experienced a major trauma but never got any help. People lauded me for initiating this discussion. Then I waited for the plan. What were we going to do? There was still time to go back and help Doris. I simply needed guidance, a course of action. But my heart sank because we did nothing but talk. A plan never materialized.

This was unfair. *Why have meetings if we aren't going to change our behavior?* I asked myself. All Doris got were antibiotics and a discharge. It was early in my medical career, but I sensed that physicians were not being trained sufficiently to address the multiple layers of health—the integration of the body, emotions, mind, and spirit. And it was at that moment that I knew I would seek a multidimensional approach to health.

And I did.

In my soul, I knew that behind every illness and symptom is a person with hurts and hopes. Even if we didn't always talk about it, I could feel it with my being. And I couldn't ignore it. My body, mind, and spirit would ache for others. Tears would well up when patients—when *people*—were sad, whether or not they said so. I couldn't focus only on the physical. It didn't make sense to me. Everything in my heart, mind, and soul steered me to see and help the *whole* person, not merely their symptoms.

After over two decades of exploration, I've learned how to help people weave the layers of health back together. It's been my life's journey. My passion. I've sought to understand health and nature by studying holistic and integrative medicine. Before starting that path, I graduated from some of the best traditional schools: Harvard, Emory, and Albert Einstein. Then, I continued to expand my perspective through a fellowship at Dr. Andrew Weil's Center for Integrative Medicine at the University of Arizona. My world opened wide, as if someone lifted a veil I had been living under. I went on to study with the Osteopathic Cranial Academy, explored the work of the medical intuitive Edgar Cayce, and became certified to teach TRE®, Tension and Trauma Release Exercises. Most importantly, I've learned to trust myself and my intuition.

If I saw someone like Doris today, I would know what to say, what to do, and especially how to *be.* At the very least, I would be present with her and acknowledge her pain. Looking her in the eye with gentleness and love, I'd let her know that no matter what she had been through, she was no less deserving of love and joy than anyone else. I would let her know I cared about her and ask if she'd like help healing an old wound.

Doris has no idea how much she impacted my perspective of medicine, health, and life. Patients like Doris have inspired me to reflect on my own life and my journey of personal growth.

Going through medical school and residency was rough on me. I would have periods when I felt down and full of self-doubt. Strangely, when I graduated from Harvard as an undergrad, I felt even more pressure to succeed. Still, I didn't trust myself and my ability to learn. By my mid-twenties, I was already burned out. I felt lost, and I had an overwhelming feeling that if I didn't make a major change, I was going to get sick.

That was my intuition knocking, and I was finally ready to listen. I started to explore my personal growth with more interest, experimenting with mind-body-spirit practices, including yoga, mindfulness, and meditation.

Through the culmination of my experiences, I've uncovered a key to healing that is not widely taught in medical training: *getting to know yourself gives you greater access to self-healing.* This includes an understanding of the true Self and our multidimensional nature—body, mind, and spirit. The answer to healing seems simple, but it's complex and elusive at the same time. Otherwise, you wouldn't be reading this book.

To understand yourself means to listen to your intuition. What is intuition exactly? It's that spark of inner guidance that comes through your body, mind, and spirit that is always loving, supportive, and encouraging. Your intuition is meant to lift you up, not bring you down, although it will give you a warning if needed. It's up to you to listen to your intuition.

I realize that the intuitive aspects of health can feel ephemeral. It's the softer side we can't always put a finger on, in contrast to the more palpable aspects of medicine, such as labs, imaging, and surgery. However, do not mistake intuition's softer side as less important or less powerful. Often, it's the intuitive part of our being that holds the most precious aspects of our lives—how we feel, connect, and love.

About This Book

I wrote this book to share with you what I've learned to help you (1) get to know yourself, (2) expand your intuitive abilities, and (3) access greater depth of healing. This book is divided into four parts: Part 1 is about the intuitive body, Part 2 the intuitive mind, and Part 3 the intuitive spirit. Part 4 will pull it all together: the intuitive human and intuitive living. The last chapter in the book is a call to action for health care.

Also, as helpful as it is to learn about intuition through reading, there's no better teacher than experience itself. This is why I've included many exercises throughout the book to give you ways to practice developing your intuition.

Developing your intuition also means fine-tuning your empathic abilities. If you're an empath, you're a "feeler" in this world. You feel things, including the emotions of those around you, the vibe of a room, the world's energy, and more (I'll go into more detail on this later). As an empath, you could also be highly sensitive about everything you feel. While there are varied definitions of what constitutes being an intuitive, an empath, and a highly sensitive person, which can be confusing, don't let the verbiage bog you down.

Here are the simple definitions I use in this book. *An intuitive* knows and understands from inner guidance. *An empath* feels emotions physically and possibly has other extrasensory abilities. *A highly sensitive person* is strongly affected by what they feel. Each type has gradients, and you can be more than one or even all three. These are also fluid, and which one(s) best describes you can change over time as you change.

Chances are, if you're holding this book, you may have an inkling that you're a feeler and would like to deepen your intuition. Those of you who are highly sensitive might discover helpful ways to process your gifts instead of getting swept away by them. And for everyone, honing your intuitive skills will deepen your connection with yourself, others, and the earth, bringing greater meaning, clarity, and joy to your life.

How to Get the Most Out of This Book

This book is meant to be used in multiple ways:

1. You can read it from beginning to end. If the concepts are relatively new to you, this would be my first recommendation.

2. Each chapter can also stand on its own, so if the subject matter is familiar, you might feel like jumping to a certain chapter. This book is meant to be a flexible resource for you.

3. In addition to the exercises in each chapter, there are bonus exercises at the end of Parts 1, 2, and 3. You don't have to do these in order; they are there to give you various ways to expand your perspective and develop your intuitive skills.

4. After you've read the book, use it as a regular resource filled with mini reminders that you are an intuitive being. You might flip through and whatever page you stop on, read it, and then do the exercise on that page or the nearest one.

5. This journey is not about being one and done. We are constantly learning throughout our lives. So, by taking an intuitive step each day, you'll add more love and joy to each moment.

PART I

The Intuitive Body

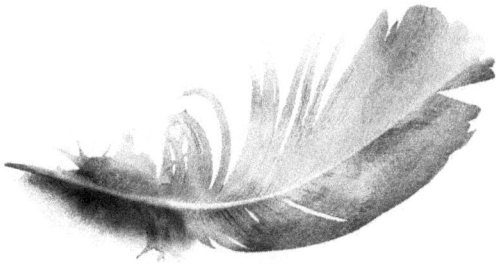

CHAPTER 1

A NEW WAY OF LOOKING AT SYMPTOMS

"Your body's symptoms are a metaphor for your life."

The first time I came across the notion that the body's symptoms are its way of communicating with us, I had to pause to let that idea settle into my understanding. I had misunderstood my body for so long. Growing up, whether I had heartburn, acne, or hay fever, I thought that meant something was wrong with me. I thought symptoms meant my body was malfunctioning and needed to be fixed, often with some kind of medication: an antacid to counter the heartburn, antibiotics for the acne, and antihistamines for the hay fever. Still, something didn't sit right because those "fixes" were only temporary. If I didn't take the antacid, my heartburn returned—so that wasn't a true healing. Sure, medications can be a lifesaver, but there are times when another way can make us feel better.

It wasn't until I learned how to redefine my body's symptoms that I also learned a different way. I didn't have to fight my body—I needed to listen and support and work with it. Looking at my body's symptoms as the body's way of speaking to me lit sparks of understanding. Did my body have a language I didn't understand? Could my symptoms hold another layer of meaning besides faulty physiology? Were the clues to feeling better already inside me? The answers are yes, yes, and yes! My understanding of health and illness was flipped entirely. The body carries an innate wisdom. If I could learn to listen to and understand my body, I could take steps toward deeper healing.

Your symptoms are speaking to you, too. They're telling you how the body is attempting to regain balance. So, how do you begin to decipher the language of the body?

Consider Your Symptoms a Metaphor for Your Life

This is your first key: consider your symptoms a metaphor for your life. Take a moment to describe your symptoms. What words or phrases come to mind? There's no right or wrong answer here because it's personal. Then, consider what areas in your life could be described with the same words metaphorically. For example, when I had reflux, I experienced a raw burning sensation that was uncomfortable and kept me up at night. I was in medical school at the time. I felt burnt out, uncomfortable with myself, and looping worries kept me up at night. That was when I found it easier to deal with the physical symptoms of reflux than to face my emotions. (More on facing our emotions in chapter 2.)

A sweet, older woman named Sally once came to me with chronic diverticulitis with ongoing abdominal pain and diarrhea. She had already been to a gastroenterologist who prescribed antibiotics, but her symptoms persisted. Sally was having difficulty digesting food. I asked her what areas in her life she also had difficulty digesting. It turned out she was the primary caretaker for her three teenage grandsons. As a mom, I knew how much energy is needed to care for kids, no matter how much we love them. I was at least a couple of decades younger than Sally, so I wondered how she was able to keep up.

I asked her, "When do you have time for yourself?"

"I don't," she told me.

Sally's number-one assignment was to do something she wanted to do every day. She didn't need any reason except that she wanted to do it. It could be sitting on the couch reading a book, calling a friend, having lunch out, whatever, as long as she chose to do it. Basically, I told her to have a little fun. In full disclosure, I also treated her osteopathically and told her to clean up her diet, but for Sally's lasting health, taking time for herself would be essential.

It was a small miracle. Sally learned how to get better. The chronic diverticulitis went away. Occasionally, it would flare after some fast food or when she wasn't taking time for herself, but the great thing was that Sally was no longer afraid of her symptoms. She understood them as a sign of what she needed to do, whether tweaking her diet or taking a break. Sally's symptoms became key to her healing because she started listening to these messages from her body. The beaming smile on her face spoke volumes about her healing.

Tensegrity—How the Body Functions as an Integrated Whole

Over time, as medicine became more and more specialized, it became harder for physicians to keep the concept of holism in mind. That's why the attending physician taking care of Doris didn't think her past trauma was relevant to her pneumonia. But now, when someone asks me if two symptoms in one person are related, my answer is typically yes! We might not know exactly how, but if the symptoms occur in one person, they are somehow connected.

Let's take a closer look at how everything in the body is related. Imagine you're holding a balloon. If you squeeze the balloon on one side, you can immediately feel the change on the other side. The body is the same way. If any pressure, tension, or other kink exists anywhere in the body, the whole body will always be affected. One of the laws of physics states that there is a reaction for every action, whether yielding or resisting. This is often referred to as *the tensegrity model*. Buckminster Fuller (1895–1983), an American architect, engineer, and inventor, coined the term *tensegrity*, combining the words *tension* and *integrity*. The balanced tension in the balloon is a perfect example of tensegrity: it resists compression by yielding as it needs to without breaking. Basically, the parts work together to strengthen the whole.

This concept of tensegrity applies to our whole being, not just the body. What affects the mind also impacts the body and vice versa. When there's a disruption to the connection to spirit, the body and mind will also reflect that disruption. Again, any one part always affects the whole. The influence might be minor, allowing a person to compensate easily, or there could be a significant impact that requires some tending but sorts out over time. There could also be small "dents" in any of the dimensions of the body, mind, or spirit, which build up over time. Some disruptions result in complete overwhelm.

How the Body Becomes Unbalanced

Stress or trauma on any of the physical, mental, emotional, or spiritual layers[1] of our being can create imbalances in the body. On the physical dimension, such stressors include injuries, environmental impacts, and nutritional needs. On the mental-emotional layers, they include feeling seen and heard, work or school stressors, grief, and betrayal. On the spiritual dimension, imbalances can result when someone doesn't experience a sense of belonging, community, or oneness. We'll be talking about each of these dimensions in further detail in each part of the book.

Whether something is stressful or traumatic depends on a person's experience. The trauma can be a big event, such as the death of a loved one, rape, or murder—but not all traumas are extreme. Trauma is any stressful incident that a person perceives as threatening their life, body, or overall well-being. In a sense, any stress can be defined as traumatic, whether big or small. Everyone experiences some trauma, and many situations you may not consider traumatic still cause significant stress. For most people, even natural life transitions such as birth and puberty can be traumatic.

Trauma is a part of life. As such, everyone's physiology has a built-in trauma response. When faced with a perceived threat, the body activates one of these stress responses—fight, flight, or freeze. (We'll get into these more later.) The body tenses, even curling into a fetal position, in preparation for one of these responses. Adrenaline and other stress hormones are released to speed up the heart rate and breathing, and our perception of time might seem to warp.

The body remembers everything that has happened in your life, everything you've thought and felt. If you have a chance to rebalance soon after a trauma, its effects might be minimal. But that doesn't always happen. If you are overwhelmed by an experience and your thoughts and feelings are not fully processed, the body holds onto them. It continues to run the physiology as if it were still experiencing the trauma. You're then living through the lens of the trauma. You may feel crazy, but you're not. What you're experiencing is *stuck physiology*, which creates an "incoordination of the nervous system."[2]

The autonomic nervous system is the part of the nervous system that does not have to be under conscious control—hence, the term *autonomic.* It has two branches: the *sympathetic* arm, responsible for the fight-or-flight response, and the *parasympathetic* arm, which is the calming or rest-and-digest aspect, as well as the freeze response. Trauma patterns in the nervous system can present in various ways, including the following.

- **Tension in the body.** When faced with overwhelming stress, to help us cope, our emotions can get tucked away in the body as tension in the tissues. But this often causes nervous system issues in the long term. Tension in the body blocks energy flow, which can occur in various degrees at many levels. It interferes with both physiology and optimal mental-emotional functioning.

- **A constant fight-or-flight response.** The nervous system can get stuck in sympathetic overload and stay in a state of fight or flight. The fight-or-flight response is a normal stress reflex that helps us in a life-threatening situation. Think of what you'd do if there were a fire inching toward you. This would create a state of high alert and anxiety. If we're in this state chronically, then everything looks like a fire or a danger to us. We may feel like running away from regular life (flight) or be aggressive or overly argumentative (fight). When we're in constant fight or flight, sleeping or thinking rationally can be difficult.

- **A constant frozen state.** When we are completely overwhelmed, the freeze response can take over due to parasympathetic overload. In this case, we can feel "spaced out" or numb. Perhaps you don't want to get out of bed or participate in daily activities. This is a protective stress response that shields us. Animals have this reflex, too; as a last resort, they play dead to avoid being eaten by a predator. The freeze response involves disassociating from the body to cope with the intensity of a danger. However, getting stuck in this state is not sustainable for overall health and well-being.

- **A mixed response.** Sometimes a traumatized person will wobble between the freeze response and the fight-or-flight response. For example, a person may go from being extremely angry and yelling to being depressed and comatose within short periods. A mixed response can also involve fawning, a behavior in which a person responds to a threat by pleasing and appeasing another while detaching from their own needs.

- **Decreased energy.** Stuck trauma also affects a person's energetic flow because it takes energy for the body to compartmentalize. There is nothing inherently wrong with tucking a trauma away—after all, this can be a helpful coping mechanism—but in the long run, it is not sustainable. Trapped energy means we no longer have access to that energy.

- **A tendency toward illness.** In addition to feeling tired, a person could feel out of balance in other ways. Their physiology won't work as well, so there could be a tendency to get sick. So, yes, Doris's past trauma did place her at more risk for illness. There is abundant research relating stress and trauma with illness. However, physicians and other healthcare practitioners aren't typically trained to get at the root of such issues.

How the Body Rebalances

Here's the good news: energy trapped by trauma can be reclaimed. The nervous system can rebalance, and the brain can change and learn. This is called *neuroplasticity*. Old patterns can be rewired to form new patterns of thought, emotions, and behavior. Some traumas lift more easily than others, of course. In general, acute traumas involving a single incident tend to shift with trauma-release therapies more quickly than chronic complex traumas and those that occurred at a younger age. Being hurt by a caretaker, loved one, or someone you trust can also leave a bigger impact.

Thankfully, humans have a remarkable capacity for resilience. Nature finds a way to grow, change, and recover. People are a part of that balance. *You* are a part of that balance and have a remarkable capacity for resilience. By releasing trauma, you can have more energy, sleep better, think more clearly, feel calmer, *and* gain more access to your intuition. Letting go of old patterns that are no longer needed helps you flow with life and maintain health and well-being.

Just as we have a built-in stress response, we also have a built-in trauma-release mechanism. These are natural reactions that allow energy and emotions to process and flow. They help to rebalance the body. Can you guess what these familiar reactions are? Let's go over various ways trauma release can naturally show up in the body.

- **Shaking.** When tension builds up, it's natural for the body to shake it off afterward. Animals do this instinctively. For example, dogs often start shaking immediately when startled by a thunderstorm. The body's shaking-off response is why dancing can be a release, too.

- **Crying.** Crying can be a healthy stress response. Tears are cleansing. Allowing ourselves to cry freely, without trying to stop the tears, can calm the nervous system.

- **Yawning.** Yes, yawning is a form of release. It encourages the body to take a deep breath.

- **Laughing.** The cliché is true: Laughing *is* one of the best medicines. It's a wonderful way to release stress, whether a nervous laugh or a full, deep-belly laugh.

- **Sighing.** When tension or confusion builds up, our body often reacts naturally with a sigh, which is a releasing breath.

- **Breathing.** All the reactions listed above encourage the body to breathe. When the breath gets stuck, so do our thoughts, emotions, and body. By encouraging the breath to calm, relax, and move freely, we can think more clearly, feel more freely, and move more easily. (More on this in chapter 2.)

Do these responses come easily to you? Or do you tend to hold them back? Do you feel like you get stuck in one of these patterns?

If you tend to feel overwhelmed, there are therapies to help you access your body's rebalancing mechanism. One of these is Tension and Trauma Release Exercises, or TRE® for short, developed by Dr. David Berceli, an international expert in trauma intervention and conflict resolution. TRE® is a set of physical exercises that help to relax the body by activating the natural shaking response. Another helpful therapy is EMDR, or Eye Movement Desensitization and Reprocessing, which uses eye movements to smooth out looping stress patterns. Another therapy called Brainspotting uses eye positions to identify and process the corresponding "brainspot" where certain thoughts and emotions are held. The Emotional Freedom Technique, also known as EFT or tapping, uses acupressure points to open up energy meridians and process stuck patterns (see page 141).

If you've suffered or suspect you've suffered severe trauma, such as abuse or violence, or if you experience PTSD (post-traumatic stress disorder), please take care to use these therapies with the help of a physician or licensed professional counselor (LPC) who is well-versed in trauma release.

The takeaway here is that your body has a natural rebalancing mechanism. If you need help, there are therapies that can support you. (See the Appendix for a list of websites and additional trauma release resources.)

These days, when I meet people in my medical practice who have been through traumatic experiences, it's no longer awkward for me. I don't shy away from the deep mental, emotional, and spiritual wounds that I know are impacting their physical health. I know how to embrace people as they are while also recognizing their healing potential. The more people can also embrace and understand themselves, the greater the opportunity for tapping into the body's intuitive and self-healing mechanisms.

So, how can you continue to get to know yourself and the language of your body? Next, let's look at the various organs and what they represent. You'll also see how stress can impact specific organs based on the emotional response triggered.

Organs and Their Emotional and Energetic Meanings

Emotions are felt through the body's physiology and interpreted by the mind. In a 2014 study published in the *Proceedings of the National Academy of Sciences*, researchers asked people to report where they felt the body sensations of certain emotions. Participants colored their answers onto what's called a body graph. The researchers found that more positive emotions like love and happiness were usually felt all over the body. They also found that the emotions we consider more negative, such as sadness and depression, caused people to feel less grounded. The negative emotions tended to be felt more in the upper body, while the positive emotions were felt all over. It seems people tend to have a more full-body presence with positive emotions. The patterns noted in this study were found across cultures.[3] In this way, emotions are a kind of universal language.

However, I find this study is oversimplified because emotions can be felt anywhere in the body. Comparing Western and Eastern medicines can provide a better understanding.

Western medicine discusses emotions in terms of the nerves and the mind, hence using more neurological terms. East Asian medicine talks about emotions in terms of more somatic and visceral functions. *Visceral* refers to the internal organs, which are associated with certain meridians, or energy channels. Emotions can have a negative impact on the organs when they get stuck or are prolonged or excessive. Health is in the flow. In other words, emotions are part of our human experience, spiritual growth, and creative expression, and we are meant to experience a rainbow of emotions.

In Eastern medicine, there are five basic emotions: grief, fear, worry, anger, and joy. Each is associated with an energy channel (or meridian) and its corresponding organ or organs.

1. **Grief** (which includes depression and sadness) corresponds to the lungs, heart, and colon.

2. **Fear** corresponds to the kidneys and bladder (also to the lungs when the kidneys are overwhelmed).

3. **Worry** (or overthinking) corresponds to the spleen, stomach, and pancreas.

4. **Anger** (which includes frustration or mania) corresponds to the liver (also to the skin when the liver is overwhelmed).

5. **Joy** corresponds to the heart.

Of course, each person's experience is unique. These are generalities, but they're also very useful generalities. If you're not sure what to do when you're feeling out of sorts, you can always start by labeling your emotions and then support your physical health by nourishing the corresponding organ. Table 1 on the next page lists ways to support the physical and energetic organ systems.

Table 1 - Ways to Support the Physical and Energetic Organ Systems

ORGAN	CORE EMOTIONS	SOME NOURISHING FOOD AND HERBS	NOURISHING ACTIVITY
Heart	Grief Joy	Cardamom Cinnamon Hawthorne tea	Opening and centering the heart field *(p. 81)* Dancing
Lungs	Grief	Mullein tea	Breathing exercises *(p. 42)* Swimming Sea salt baths
Spleen	Worry	Astragalus root in soups and broths	Walking Dance organically *(p. 80)*
Stomach	Worry	Chamomile tea Digestive bitters	Walking Humming for vagal toning *(p. 76)*
Pancreas	Worry	Digestive bitters Probiotic foods and drinks	Walking Belly breathing *(p. 43)*
Liver *(Skin is also related)*	Anger	Apple cider vinegar (a spoonful) Digestive bitters	Walking Letting your scream out *(p. 110)*
Kidney *(Lungs and adrenals are also related)*	Fear Grief	Dandelion greens Staying hydrated	Walking Sea salt bath Naming all your emotions Add color to life *(p. 189)*
Bladder	Fear	Gotu kola Staying hydrated	Add color to life *(p. 189)*

On the flip side, if you have physical symptoms and are having trouble addressing them, consider how the corresponding core emotions might apply. These are stepping-stones that give you ideas on what steps to take toward better health. They are direct messages from your body, so learning the body's language is worthwhile.

Remember my patient Doris, who had pneumonia? From the table, you can see that the unprocessed grief and fear from her rape could have affected the function of her lungs. Do you see how understanding the organs and their corresponding core emotions can help expand our ideas on healing?

Integrating the Body with Cross-Lateral Exercises

Of course, the organs do not function on their own. It's also important to help integrate the body as a whole. To function well, both the right and left sides of the body and brain need to be integrated, meaning they must communicate. Typically, when the body and mind are not functioning optimally, the signals between the two sides of the brain could use help flowing more freely. Imagine a traffic jam versus cars moving freely on a highway. We need both hemispheres to work together to coordinate movement, learn new things, feel calm, and have energy. Otherwise, it's as if the body is functioning on half a battery.[4]

Signals from each brain hemisphere cross to the other side via the corpus callosum. So, how can we help the brain signals integrate? Abundant research shows that cross-lateral (cross-body) movements help the right and left brain hemispheres connect and coordinate. According to neurophysiologist Dr. Carla Hannaford, "Cross-lateral movements, like a baby's crawling, activate both hemispheres in a balanced way . . . When both eyes, both ears, both hands and feet are being used equally, the corpus callosum orchestrating these processes between the two hemispheres becomes more fully developed."[5]

Cross-body movements can help

- Relax tension
- Improve coordination
- Calm the mind
- Boost energy and endurance
- Increase focus and fluid thinking

Whether you need to discharge or recharge your batteries, cross-body movements can help. I've seen kids improve their handwriting after a month or two by doing these exercises, which can also help with athletic abilities (for repeated injuries) and innovative thinking (before a presentation or a test). Give it a try with this simple exercise, which takes just a few minutes a day.

Exercise: The Cross-Lateral March

Cross-lateral movements are meant to be natural movements like walking, crawling, or dancing, helping the body to reset regularly. Stand with feet hip-distance apart. Now, do an exaggerated march in place or across the floor. As you raise your left knee, bring your right hand over to touch it. As you raise your right knee, bring your left hand over to touch it. Do this twice daily for 1 to 2 minutes or 10 to 20 repetitions.

Take note if there's difficulty crossing the midline—for example if the right hand keeps going to the right knee or the left hand to the left knee. If you're helping a child having a hard time with the cross-lateral movements, help with the movements until the child can do it on their own.

There are also many variations and modifications of this exercise:

- Cross-march while sitting: Do the same movements as above but while sitting down.

- Cross-crawl: It's how babies crawl! The right arm moves with the left leg, and the left arm moves with the right leg. The cross-crawl is often done with post-stroke patients during rehabilitation.

- Windmills: While standing, touch right hand to left foot and then left hand to right foot.

- Many yoga poses, such as the Eagle, Tabletop Balance, and spinal twists, engage cross-lateral movements.

(See page 75 for other cross-lateral exercises.)

There's more to understand about integrating the left and right sides of the body. Our left and right sides respectively represent the feminine and masculine energies. Let's explore this in more detail because there's a wealth of wisdom in understanding the feminine and masculine energies.

Feminine and Masculine Energies

First, I need to clarify that the concept of masculine and feminine energies is not based on gender. We all have masculine and feminine energies; when they are balanced, we feel whole—more alive and more like ourselves. Naturally, we all have different constitutions. Some people have more masculine energies, and others have more feminine energies. Generally, females tend to have more feminine energy and males tend to have more masculine energy, but this is completely fluid. As we know, gender itself is a fluid construct, and these energies are as well.

Looking at the Chinese symbols of yin and yang can help us better understand the fluidity of these energies.

Figure 1 - Yin-Yang

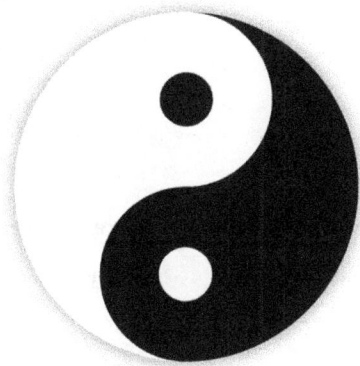

Yin-Yang

The yin-yang is a symbol of Taoism, a philosophy based on the teachings of Lao Tzu, a sixth-century BC sage. (I love philosophy, which I find so helpful in healing.) The yin-yang symbol has two similar parts that both flow into each other. If you imagine the symbol rotating like fishes swimming in a circle, each "fish" flows into the other. So, this is not a strict, black-and-white concept. It is fluid and ever-changing. Plus, the meanings of what is yin and what is yang are relative to each other, which is represented by the two dots in the symbol. In other words, there are aspects of the masculine in the feminine and aspects of the feminine in the masculine. Even though we can list masculine versus feminine energetic properties, these are not strict delineations. However, this list does give us a framework for discussion.

Yin is the feminine, and yang is the masculine. Similarly, the moon at night is considered feminine, while the sun in the day is considered masculine. The sun and the moon are a perfect example of how each flows into the other. Night flows into the day, and day flows into the night. Also, the feminine is considered more receptive and nourishing, while the masculine is more active and providing. You can see how their characteristics are similar yet different. This table highlights other yin and yang characteristics:

Table 2 – Feminine (Yin) and Masculine (Yang) Energies

FEMININE (YIN)	MASCULINE (YANG)
LEFT side of the body	RIGHT side of the body
Moon / night	Sun / day
More receptive	More giving
More nurturing	More providing
More yielding	More assertive
More creative and innovative	More stable and steady
Strength in vulnerability	Strength in confidence
More flowing and intuitive	More logical and analytical
More authentic	More honest
More fluid boundaries	More rigid boundaries
Protective	
Supportive	
Caring	

When we look at the body, the left side tends to be more feminine, while the right side tends to be more masculine. Keep in mind that most of the nerve signals from one side of the brain cross to direct the opposite side of the body. That means that the feminine/left side of the body is more "right-brained," and the masculine/right side is more "left-brained." You can see why cross-lateral exercises would help integrate and balance our yin-yang energies.

Remember: we are all made up of both yin and yang. It's about balance. Understanding the balance (or imbalance) of masculine and feminine energies can help us interpret messages from the body. For instance, after my dad passed, I had an achiness in my right shoulder, and strangely, my sister had pain in her right shoulder. Again, the right side of the body is more masculine, so this could represent relationships with male figures in our lives. It was easy for me to make sense of this ache as it related to my dad's crossing over.

On the other hand, I had a patient with right-sided shoulder pain that had to do with her mother, as it was related to an argument she had with her mother over money. Finances tend to be the domain of the masculine. The moment she made the connection and processed those emotions, her pain lifted.

These examples also show how feminine and masculine energies are not hardline constructs. They are fluid. The yin-yang concepts are useful for feeling, hearing, and listening to the body's stories. Having the foundations and vocabulary to organize and describe what you're feeling helps you understand yourself on many different dimensions, which helps you feel more whole. Another way to get more attuned to your masculine and feminine energies would be with the exercise on page 78: A Conversation with Your Masculine and Feminine Energies.

Exercise: What Is Your Body Saying to You?
We've gone through many ways that your body communicates to you:

- Using your symptoms as metaphors
- Organs and their energetic meaning
- Left-sided (feminine) and right-sided (masculine) symptoms

Now, you'll start writing the story of your body. What are your body's symptoms? What are they saying to you? Where in your life do you feel the metaphor of your body's symptoms or vice versa? Where in your body do you feel the challenges and joys in your life? Use the tables in this chapter to help you interpret your body's language. Understanding your body is a big part of healing. You might also choose to express love and thanks for your body; for guidance on that, check out this exercise: Writing a Letter to Your Body on page 77.

Summary

Your body's symptoms are a metaphor for your life. They are messages from the body to your intuition showing you where the healing is. In this chapter, we covered

- Symptoms as metaphor
- Tensegrity—how you are a whole human being, and what affects one part also affects the whole
- Stress and trauma on any dimension of our being (physical, mental, emotional, spiritual) creating imbalance(s) in the body
- The body's natural rebalancing mechanisms
- How the organs correspond to core emotions
- How integrating the right and left sides of the body and brain helps you feel more whole
- How the left and right sides of the body also correspond to feminine and masculine energies

* * *

Do you find that some parts of your story are more difficult to look at? Most people do. You might have a heart shield up, making it difficult to dive in and heal more deeply. In the next chapter, we'll look at the heart to further your understanding of the intuitive body.

CHAPTER 2

GROUNDING THE BODY
AND OPENING THE HEART

"When we ground, we let built-up energy discharge into the ground—in the same way that an electrical circuit needs to be grounded for stability to prevent electrical shock."

I wasn't always grounded. I was hesitant and shy for at least the first couple of decades of my life. I was anxious about most things, though I'd try to hide it. Sometimes, I could hide it, but not always. Other times, I looked like a deer in headlights. That doesn't mean I didn't accomplish much because I did—it's that I wasn't fully present in my body. I tended to be more in my head. Typically, I could still feel my heart, too, but I was confused. I didn't know what part of myself to listen to, the analytical me or the dreamer. It was a constant battle, so I didn't make decisions easily. In the extreme, I would be more dissociated. I could daydream easily, especially when I was sad, frustrated, or bored. Occasionally, when my teachers would call on me, I had no idea what they were talking about because I was caught up in my daydream.

When you're that out of touch with reality, you're less likely to make healthy decisions. Because I wasn't fully connected to my body, I didn't hear my body's messages. I tended to overeat. I thought it was normal to feel so full and for my belly to hurt afterward. I also pushed myself past the limit of being tired. Then, I would oversleep to compensate and repeat the cycle again and again.

I didn't know it then, but I needed to ground myself. I needed to settle into my body to have more clarity and learn to trust myself. I needed to listen to my body and regain access to my intuition.

What Does It Mean to Be Grounded?

When we're thinking intensely, the electrical activity in the brain increases, and it builds up a charge. Have you noticed that when you're studying or thinking hard, there's more tension in your neck and head? That's because energy is rising to your brain. The same thing happens when we're stressed. When we ground, we let that built-up energy discharge into the ground—in the same way that every electrical circuit needs to be grounded for stability to prevent electrical shock.

We are made up of energy—everything is. In physics, we learn that energy is the measurement of the potential to do work or cause change. The human body has different types of energy, including the ones listed in this table:

Table 3 - Types of Energy

TYPE OF ENERGY	DEFINITION	EXAMPLE
Chemical	The energy stored in chemical bonds	The energy released when breaking down molecules of food
Elastic	The energy stored in objects under tension	Tendons can act like springs when running
Thermal	The energy from heat	Helps to maintain a constant body temperature
Kinetic	The energy from motion	Helps us to move
Electrical	The energy from the movement of electrons in atoms	Nerve impulses
Electromagnetic	Radiant energy that travels at the speed of light	The heart field

When it comes to grounding the body, we tend to focus only on its electrical energy, but all its forms of energy are related. Remember that energy cannot be created or destroyed, but it can be transformed from one type of energy to another.

The following table lists some of the common signs of both being ungrounded and grounded:

Table 4 - Signs of Being Ungrounded vs Grounded

	SIGNS OF BEING UNGROUNDED	SIGNS OF BEING GROUNDED
Body	Not paying attention to the body's messages: overeating; overdrinking; forgetting to eat, drink, pee, sleep, or exercise; out of touch with nature	Listening to the body's messages: eating just enough and regularly; staying hydrated; getting adequate sleep and exercise; connecting with and appreciating nature
Emotions	Overwhelmed with emotion; numbing emotion; clinging to good times and pushing difficult times away	Allowing uncomfortable emotions to be and processing them; living in the moment and appreciating joyful times while able to experience difficult times and then let them go
Mind	Lost in thought; looping thoughts; overthinking or overanalyzing; indecision; not in the flow; daydreaming or feeling spacey; anxiety; procrastinating; staying overbusy; choosing activities or behaviors that create an adrenaline rush; mania	Fluid thoughts; more innovation and creativity; being in the flow; balancing rest and play; mindful presence
Spirit	Limited access to intuition, if any; not seeing the beauty in life; not living fully; ignoring self-care; depression; having difficulty bringing the calm of meditation into the rest of life	More access to intuition; following life's guidance; seeing beauty even in the mundane; appreciating time alone to reset; prioritizing self-care

Being grounded is a gradient, not an all-or-nothing state. It's a gradient from ungrounded to grounded. When you are completely grounded, you are fully present in your body. When you are completely ungrounded, that's a total dissociative state, where you are completely out of touch with reality or frozen or comatose in a state of depression. When we're ungrounded, we don't feel entirely like ourselves and won't live to our potential.

Once I became more grounded, I felt less rushed about things. I could be calmer and think clearly, even in chaos. I began to eat just the right amount of food, no overeating or undereating. And once I became more grounded, my intuition opened, bringing me a whole new world.

In this chapter, we will look at grounding the body, the heart, and the emotions.

What Makes It Difficult to Ground?

Many forms of distraction can draw your presence away from yourself. Here are some that you can choose to shift:

1. Eating an unbalanced and nutrient-deprived diet.

You want your food to be filled with nourishing nutrients and high vibes. A nutrient-deprived diet is high in sugar, processed foods, sodas, caffeine, and alcohol. All these innutritious foods and drinks numb our connection with the body. Artificial food additives do the same thing and include synthetic chemicals, food dyes, and preservatives. If you eat animal products, it's important to consider how the animals have been treated and the quality of food they've been fed. Many foods are laden with pesticides, including those fed to animals. In general, when it's not good for the earth, it's not good for us.

Although chemicals in food are not healthy for anyone, some people are more sensitive to them than others. If you are one of those people, these chemicals can feel like a wrench has been thrown into your nervous system. You could feel irritable, anxious, hyperactive, have trouble concentrating, and feel ungrounded. Your body could also show signs of inflammation, such as rashes, a stuffy nose, or digestive issues.

Europe has banned chemicals in foods that the United States continues to use regularly, such as potassium bromate in breads and pastries and brominated vegetable oil in citrus-flavored soft drinks.[1] The Environmental Working Group is a nonprofit highlighting outdated legislation, harmful agricultural practices, and industry loopholes that pose a risk to our health and our environment.[2] According to the EWG, the following non-organic foods made the Dirty Dozen in their 2023 list, which means they contain the most pesticides: strawberries; spinach; kale, collard, and mustard greens; peaches; pears; nectarines; apples; grapes; bell and hot peppers; cherries; blueberries; and green beans.[3]

An imbalanced diet can be addictive, so you may find it challenging to change your diet. Keep in mind, though, that addressing your diet doesn't have to be an all-or-nothing endeavor. Take small steps every day toward eating a clean and balanced diet. If you are struggling, see an integrative physician first to make sure there aren't any urgent medical issues. Then, consider working with a wellness coach or a food support group. (More resources are listed at the end of the book.)

For a quick summary, here are the basics of eating clean and avoiding nerve irritants:

- Buy organic from the Dirty Dozen to decrease the pesticides you eat.
- Avoid artificial dyes and artificial preservatives.
- Decrease or avoid caffeine.
- Decrease or avoid alcohol.
- Decrease or avoid sugar.
- Eat a (mostly) plant-based diet with plenty of greens.[4]

One of the greatest benefits of clean eating is that it becomes easier to eat intuitively. What is intuitive eating? It's when you can look at different foods and know what your body needs. When we eat a lot of junk, it puts both the brain and the body in a fog. We don't think and process things as efficiently. You may not even realize this if you've always eaten this way. But when the fog lifts, it will be a whole new world.

This happened to my brother Jojo after he hit rock bottom with his health. His body was so inflamed that he itched constantly and had painful rashes; he was bloated and overweight, and he had chronic asthma. He was barely hanging on, yet a tiny spark within urged him onward. Jojo sought a better understanding of his health issues and turned to the integrative health field for answers. Addressing his diet was a major turning point, but it wasn't easy. So, he focused on small successes as he slowly changed his diet. It took him a year to cut out all the sugar and junk food without having any detox reactions. He remembers how good the junk food tasted but no longer craves it. The food no longer controls him. And a bonus for Jojo is having so much more access to his intuition. Now, he can walk through a buffet line and know which foods his body needs. He's also found that he's more intuitive in social interactions. He picks up on subtle emotional cues, like if a co-worker hopes to talk to him about a family issue that isn't work-related. Before, Jojo might have missed such a cue. Clean eating isn't just about food and nutrition; it's also about how food makes us feel and can help us harmonize our mind, body, and spirit to tap into our super senses.

2. Chaotic energy in your environment.
Take a look at your environment. We are an overstimulated society, bombarded with information. As you align your body, mind, and spirit, you'll find you need regular quiet and calm in your life to rebalance and ground. Then, you're more equipped to face life's challenges. It's impossible to feel whole while running on empty. So, how can you create an environment that is soothing and nourishing? It's not about controlling your entire environment but creating a nourishing space. Even a small space in your home can be a haven.

To create a nourishing nest for yourself, consider your physical senses: sight, sound, smell, touch, and taste. What is in your visual environment? Is the television often on? Do you find yourself looking at your phone for much of the day? Does your space feel cluttered? See if you can reduce visual distractions by organizing your environment and spending digital time wisely. Are there colors you're drawn to? What kinds of sounds are in your space? What difference would playing soothing music make? What about the scents in your environment? Is the air fresh, or does the room need to be aired? You might choose to infuse the atmosphere with the scent of gentle essential oils. Scents are personal, and not everyone wants added aromas. Avoid artificial scents because, like the chemicals in foods, artificial scents can irritate the body. What sorts of textures surround you? Do they feel welcoming? Are you wearing comfortable clothes? During the pandemic, when we were home on lockdown, more people chose soft, cozy clothing they could easily move in. And what sorts of flavors are you eating, and are the foods you choose nourishing?

We can use nature as a model for creating our safe haven. Think of a beautiful scene in nature. What sorts of sensory input does it provide? The elements of water, wind, earth, and fire have multisensory aspects. Is there a way to represent more than one element in your space? Make your haven personal to you.

You'll discover that when you've cleared the energy in your environment, there will be less static in your subtle energy body and more space for you to ground into your body. I'll discuss the subtle energy body in more detail in the next chapter.

3. Spending too much time indoors.
When we spend too much time indoors, static charge builds up in the body. That charge literally needs to ground into the earth. Getting out in nature helps us to discharge and reset. We are meant to interact with nature. Studies have shown that regularly grounding in nature helps to keep the heart open, regulates blood pressure, soothes nerves, and boosts the immune system.[5,6] In the 1980s in Japan, the term *shinrin-yoku*, or "forest bathing," emerged with a new emphasis on the therapeutic benefits of taking nature in with our senses.

Here are some ideas for ways to take in nature:
- Go for a walk.
- Rest your back against a tree.
- Go barefooted on the ground.
- Sit or lie down on the ground.
- Dance in the rain.
- Watch the sun rise or set.

- Look for constellations.
- Listen to the birds.
- Swim in a lake, ocean, or other natural body of water.
- Build fairy houses.
- Gather sticks.
- Make a rock tower.
- Plant a garden.

When you can't get out into nature, research has found that just looking at nature photos is also beneficial for your health.[7]

4. Generational trauma.

Sometimes, the intensity of uncomfortable symptoms can feel bigger than you. Such symptoms can be triggers and patterns passed down through the generations in your family—from your parents, grandparents, great-grandparents, etc. You may or may not be aware of the stressors or traumas they experienced, but your cells know. Generational trauma is real.

There can be variations in gene expression—*epigenetics* is a whole field of science dedicated to understanding how gene expression changes with our behavior and environment. According to epigenetics, it's not that a genetic code is changed but *how* that code is interpreted. Our cells can read and interpret the same set of genes in different ways.

Some initial studies that launched the epigenetics field looked at the consequences of the Dutch Famine Winter on pregnant women and their babies during World War II. The studies found that by middle age, those children had higher rates of obesity, cardiovascular disease, diabetes, and schizophrenia.[8] These children were born stressed. When we're stressed, we're not grounded. If you've been in a stressed state all your life, it can be difficult to notice that you're in one. An understanding of generational trauma can help. Understanding that your life is more than your life alone helps you understand yourself, your story, and what came before you, the story you were born into.

Your body holds the wisdom of your history. When you can see how certain patterns formed, you can choose to change them. Your genes do not seal your fate. You can change the way your genes are expressed.[9] How? There are many ways, from making healthy food choices to decreasing your exposure to pollutants, incorporating regular exercise, making room for rest and rejuvenation, and shifting your thoughts and perceptions. In other words, reducing stress through overall grounding can influence your gene expression. We'll be discussing what helps you ground throughout this book. In short, both your compassionate understanding of yourself and others and being kind and nurturing to yourself and others will help to ground you. You can create a ripple effect for generations to come.

5. Resisting emotional challenges—the heart shield.

When we feel the need to protect our heart, we often become guarded and ungrounded. It's a coping mechanism to shield ourselves. This is a common state for many people, especially when life is overwhelming. By not being fully in the body, they also don't have to be fully present to their challenges. But if we desire to live fully, we have to face our difficulties at some point.

A *heart shield* is particularly important to address because it will block the communication of the heart, and we are meant to be heart-centered beings. The heart's messages are sent out in multiple ways throughout the body, including through nerve impulses, hormones and neurotransmitters, pressure waves, sound waves, light waves, and electromagnetic waves. According to research from the Institute of HeartMath, the heart's electrical field is about 60 times greater than that of the brain, and the heart's magnetic field is more than 100 times greater than the brain's. Let's explore the concept of the heart shield more through Mark's story.

Mark had been having heart palpitations for several months. He also felt like he had a weight on his shoulders and chest. These heart-related symptoms scared him, so he went to a cardiologist for a full workup, only to be told everything was normal. He didn't have a heart attack, there were no dangerous arrhythmias noted, and an echocardiogram showed that the heart muscles and valves were functioning well. That was all good news, but Mark still didn't know what was causing the sensations in his heart.

He had been under a lot of stress as the dad of three young kids and the financial provider for his family during the pandemic. When he met with me, he admitted to feeling anxious and worried most of the time. I found a lot of tension in his body. His shoulders were slightly rounded, though not noticeable unless you're really looking. His core muscles and the muscles in his chest were tense. Mark was smiling, but there were worry lines on his forehead. I understood that all that tension could be putting some physical pressure on his heart, as well as the nerves going to and from the heart.

Fortunately, osteopathic treatment helped to rebalance Mark's autonomic nervous system, calming the fight-or-flight response, boosting the relaxation response, and easing the tension in his body. For his homework, I gave him a few physical exercises to help release the tension in his shoulders, chest, and core. I also asked him to incorporate some of the mind-body exercises I share in this book. Within just a week, Mark's heart palpitations and feelings of panic subsided.

Can you start to see the story of Mark's symptoms? The pressure in his life was mirrored by the pressure in his body and the symptoms he felt. Because of the overwhelm in his life, Mark had put up what I call "heart shield," a form of protection, a kind of armor, which keeps us from feeling another life sting. It's a way to get through difficult times, and because life can be hard, many people have, to some degree, put up a heart shield.

However, there is a price to the heart shield.

1. When we carry armor, there's a heaviness to it. You could notice this as a weight on your neck, chest, and shoulders; as a tension headache; a curling in of the body and core muscles; or a lack of depth in your breath.

2. There can be cardiac symptoms with or without a known cause. (If you have cardiac symptoms, please consult a cardiologist or other qualified physician even if the heart shield is a component because it's important to address all layers of your being.)

3. The heart shield can prevent you from feeling the depths of joy and happiness because the shield works to block feelings, whether hurt or joy. So we can't experience life fully when we've put up a heart shield.

4. Because of the shield, your connection to yourself and others is limited, which leads us to the fifth cost:

5. Limited connection also limits full access to your intuition.

Putting the heart shield down takes courage. This is about vulnerability. Brene´ Brown sums this up when she says, "Vulnerability is the birthplace of connection." It is hard enough for anyone to feel vulnerable, so for you to *choose* vulnerability takes some mega-insight.

Let's quickly review: Stress creates tension in the body and curls the body up toward the fetal position. People who are depressed will be well aware of this caving-in sensation. Once we're out of the womb, we're meant to uncurl. It's interesting to note that in the fetus's development, the face uncurls from the heart. Your facial expression is meant to show what the heart feels. With stuck emotions, however, this is less likely to occur because the subtle energy field of the face will be curled in toward the heart, like an ostrich with its head in the sand (more on this in chapter 3). Curled-up stress is commonly felt in the hips, the core muscles, the shoulders, the neck, and anywhere else. The tension in the body can also place pressure on the heart and cause palpitations and other cardiovascular issues. Uncurling the heart and lifting the heart shield are vital for multidimensional health. Here are a few exercises to help you with this.

Exercise: Lowering the Heart Shield
First, I hope for you to understand that lowering the heart shield will take checking in regularly with yourself. Your heart shield goes up and down naturally, depending on your response to life. The goal is not to put it down and keep it down; instead, this is a practice of working with the heart shield, a way of living.

When you become aware that you need to lower your shield, begin by acknowledging how it has helped you. Breathe this recognition in— really feel this in your body. You've made it this far, and that's a lot. You could place your hands over your heart as you do this to help bring your awareness there. Then, consider whether you would like to feel even more love, happiness, and joy in your life. How might shielding yourself now no longer serve you the way it did? Give thanks for how it has helped, and tell yourself that it's okay now to lower the heart shield.

Slowly, bit by bit, as your heart is ready. Doing this may feel raw and awkward because you may become more aware of some uncomfortable emotions. We'll address this later in this chapter.

Exercise: Opening Up Your Wings

I have recommended this exercise to so many patients. It helps them round back the shoulders, lift the heart, and open up the back of the heart. It's a simple exercise of imagination that directs healing energy to lift and lower the heart shield:

1. Imagine the area between your shoulder blades where wings would sprout.

2. See your wings sprout and grow.

3. Now imagine them opening up completely on both sides.

4. Feel the extra support as they lift and uncurl your heart.

I had a patient I'll call Sandy. She was a teacher who had chronic tension in her chest because of ongoing stress from her job. After I helped her open up her thorax with osteopathic treatment, I gave her this opening-up-your-wings exercise to add to her self-care routine. The first time she tried it was with me, and I could immediately see Sandy's wilted stance and rounded shoulders unfurl with confidence and more joy. Whenever she feels stressed at work, Sandy now gives herself mini boosts throughout the day by imagining her wings opening. Facing her day is no longer overwhelming because she knows how to care for herself regularly; she doesn't let the constant stress pile up. Sandy also told her friends and colleagues about this exercise to help them through their stressful days.

You will find additional exercises to help you reconnect with your heart and lower the heart shield at the end of Part 1. Don't feel you have to do them all. Start with the ones that feel easier for you. If you've had a heart shield up for a while, remember to be gentle, and when it's difficult to deal with emotions head-on, take a break. Go to the physical body and create flow by moving your body, which we'll look at in the next section.

Grounding Through Mindful Movement

In chapter 1, we discussed how tension in your body can hold stuck emotions. Movement helps by easing tension and relaxing the body. As your body unfolds in movement, the emotions can be released, processed, and grounded. The word *emotion* was derived from the French word *émotion*, which means "a physical disturbance." Our "e-motions" naturally want to move and process; "motion" is built into the word. It's amazing how language itself can hold clues to health. The clue here is that health is found in the flow. You can move your body to help process your emotions—the trick is to do so with awareness.

Movement is meant to be joyful. When toddlers learn to walk, they are motivated and delighted. They fall over, and then they get back up, again and again. To help you become more aware of your body, check out the Progressive Muscle Relaxation exercise on page 79, and for some direction with the joyful movement of dance, see Dancing Organically on page 80.

This next exercise will have you explore the relationship between your posture, your heart, and your breath.

Exercise: Breathing to Feel the Neutral Heart and the Folded Heart

To feel the difference, you will compare your breathing in a more neutral posture with a rounded one:

- First, stand straight up, rolling your shoulders back and down for a neutral posture, and let your chest be nice and open. Think of how a superhero would stand with a relaxed confidence. Be careful not to exaggerate the chest opening and puff it out. Let it be open with neutral ease. Take a few minutes to breathe in this position. How does your heart feel? How do your lungs feel?

- Then, see what it feels like to hunch your shoulders over and curl in on your heart and lungs. Take a few breaths there for comparison. What does your heart feel like now? How about your lungs?

The effects are more than just physical. Your heart field can also feel dampened and pulled inward. It can feel like a veil has been placed over the light of your heart.

If you don't have great posture, there's no need to get down about it. That tension in your body serves as a reminder to uncurl it. The body will mold into whatever position it's used to. Your body also hopes to protect you, so it will automatically curl in if you feel stressed. It's your body helping you, even if you don't realize it. But once you notice you're curled in, you can talk to your body to let it know whether you still need to be in this position.

When I'm tired, my body is more likely to curl in. I also noticed this when recovering from giving birth; I felt exhausted and vulnerable, much like my newborn. My body curled in again the first six months after my dad crossed over. During those months, I felt raw and beat up in a different way. In these extreme moments, it was much more apparent to me. My body was talking to me, telling me to rest and take care. When I'm aware of it, I can prioritize more time to move, stretch, do yoga, rest, and let myself be until I feel safe to uncurl again.

Understanding Your Breath and How It Helps You to Ground
The breath is always affected when we are stressed, and how we breathe indicates how connected we are to the body. By understanding various breathing patterns, you can use breathwork to help yourself ground. Here are some common breathing patterns I see when people are stressed:

1. Holding the breath
Many people have a "catch" in their breath. They may seem fine outwardly, but the breath doesn't move freely from in-breath to out-breath. Even when directed to take a deep breath consciously, a "catch" remains in their breathing, with increased tension as they try to inhale deeply. Breathing also tends to be higher in those with a catch, more in the chest than in the belly. It can also feel difficult to let go and exhale completely. A nervous tension keeps things in as if slightly holding the breath could control the stress or make it disappear. This can also be a bit of subconscious numbing of stuck emotions—in other words, "If I don't acknowledge those emotions, maybe they don't exist." Also, an incomplete inhalation is an insufficient stress response; in this case, you're not responding with your full breath or ability. If you notice

yourself holding your breath, use a gentle awareness to encourage more movement in the breath.

2. Shallow breathing

In shallow breathing, a person is breathing high into the chest. There doesn't seem to be depth. This goes hand in hand with holding your breath. There are many different types of breathing; a small breath can still be efficient if the body has a good flow. However, most people I see with shallow breathing have a lot of tension in their bodies. In that case, allow yourself to take slow, calm, deep breaths to help calm the body.

3. Breathing fast, even at rest

Many people are chronically hyperventilating but don't realize it. An increased respiratory rate is a natural part of the stress response. However, if you're chronically stressed, you're probably blowing off too much carbon dioxide, which could make the body a bit more acidic, leading to dizziness, fatigue, insomnia, and confusion, all of which could lead to more stress. It becomes a self-perpetuated cycle. So, see if you can slow down your breathing in a way that still feels comfortable. Again, be gentle. More is not necessarily better; neither is pushing yourself too hard.

4. Forced deep breathing

As you notice your breath, be gentle and follow the ease. There's a tendency for the mind to want to be pushy, and then breathing starts to feel more mechanical, like a robot's. This happened to me when I first started yoga. I so wanted to do the breathwork right, but my breath ended up being forced and machine-like. I had to remind myself to lighten up and find the balance between making an effort and not trying too hard.

When we are grounded, breathing has an ease to its rhythms. There is no forced inhalation or exhalation, and the rate is calm. Breathwork can help us maintain a sense of peace and rebalance when we're stressed. I love breathwork because it's a kind of meditation. When you're new to meditation, it can be intimidating for some. Bringing awareness to the breath is a great place to start. And even when we're more experienced at meditation, there is still a lifetime of depth to get out of breathwork.

In general, what you need to know about the breath is that inhalation encourages the sympathetic nervous system (fight or flight), and exhalation encourages the parasympathetic nervous system (rest and digest). To feel grounded, we need the sympathetic and parasympathetic parts of the nervous system to be in balance.

Table 5 - Inhalation vs Exhalation

INHALATION the in-breath	EXHALATION the out-breath
Encourages the sympathetic nervous system (We need oxygen for fight or flight.)	Encourages the parasympathetic nervous system (We need to let go to rest and digest.)
Increases heart rate	Decreases heart rate
Energizing	Calming

Breathing Exercises

You can use the breath to change your nervous system's response. What follows are some breathing exercises to do this. The timing and ratio of both the inhalation and exhalation matter. Many breathing exercises promote calm by focusing on moving your breath, slowing your breathing, and extending the exhalation.

The Long Exhale

One of the first breathing exercises I teach people is the extended exhale. Breathe in slowly through your nose and then exhale slowly through your mouth, as if you were blowing a candle flame without blowing it out. See if you can exhale at least twice as long as you inhale. Singers use a long exhale to hold a long note. One of my patients was feeling anxious about an upcoming sports tournament. Her heart was racing, and she felt dizzy and nauseated. She was able to learn how to calm herself with the long exhale. After a few minutes, her heart was no longer racing, and she felt more relaxed. The dizziness and nausea also diffused. She was able to use the long exhale to calm feelings of panic. Even four to five breaths like this can make a difference.

Belly Breathing

Have you ever noticed how little children tend to stand and breathe? Their posture shows confidence: the belly is relaxed and out, and the chest is unfolded, not tense. They are in love with themselves and the world around them. Then stuff happens, and children and their breathing start to curl up. Let belly breathing be a simple reminder to you to stand tall. To practice, move the breath gently—do not force— and as you inhale, let your belly expand outward and your diaphragm muscle expand downward. Your diaphragm is just under the lungs. On the exhalation, let the belly naturally draw inward as air moves out of the lungs and the diaphragm rounds upward again. The diaphragm relaxes on the exhale, so see if you can let go and exhale just a little bit more than usual. Belly breathing promotes lung function, allowing stagnant air to be expelled and increasing oxygen exchange.

The Space Between Breaths

The space between breaths is that natural pause at the top of an inhalation and again at the bottom of the exhalation. The space between breaths doesn't get as much attention as inhaling and exhaling, but it is full of potential. The space between breaths holds the ever-present peace in the universe—there is stillness even in chaos.

To work with the space between breaths:

- Bring your gentle attention to your breathing.
- Give yourself some time to settle in, and then listen to the space between breaths.
- Let your awareness linger until your breathing naturally wants to move to the next part of the breath.

You might notice that your breathing starts to calm, with tension easing out simply by allowing. (This breathing practice would be great to combine with the mindful exercise Finding Stillness in the Storm on page 137.)

You Are 99.999 Percent Space

Let's do a tiny review of matter and what we are made of. We are made of atoms. Each atom has a central nucleus containing protons and neutrons. The nucleus is surrounded by an electron cloud. That electron cloud is a *potential* cloud since the electron cannot be everywhere at once. If we were to scale this model with the nucleus being the size of a pea, then the surrounding electron cloud would be the size of a baseball stadium. Imagine that—a pea in the middle of a baseball stadium! That's a lot of potential space there. Again, the electron(s) cannot be everywhere at once, so the potential cloud is also potential space.

That's exactly where the wiggle room is. Space is a neutral void until you fill it with something. What exactly could you fill the space in your body with? Your awareness! You can fill the space with your awareness by breathing into it. So, let's try that now.

Take a big breath and sigh it out. Shake out any jitters and settle into your body. Then, gently bring your breath to the space between all your body's cells. In this space is the neutrality of nothingness. There are no illusions in this space, only endless possibilities. In this space is omni-potential, the limitless potential from which all things arise. Nothing has been created yet in this space. Take some slow, gentle, deep breaths into this space-between-things, and appreciate its neutrality. Breathe into the infinite potential and appreciate that it's not part of the illusion. We get to create in this space, we get to be in this space, we get to live in this space; but first, we must notice it. With your breath, breathe into the space between each cell; then breathe into the space between each atom; then breathe into the space of each atom, including the potential cloud space where the electrons aren't. Nothing is tugging at you in this space. Everything just is. You can just be. You get to create from this space, because from here anything is possible. Practice breathing in that spaciousness.

The body communicates with us through the breath. If you ignore your breathing, your body's messages will keep getting stronger until you can't help but notice. How does your body send messages? Through discomfort and symptoms. The sooner you pay attention to your breath and body, the smoother your path will become.

You can also use your breath to move through any symptoms you might have, whether physical, mental, emotional, or spiritual. Your breath can help you flow through life. Combining your breath with self-awareness is like giving a hug to whatever part of yourself you focus on.

Exploring Emotions and Grounding— The Avocado and the Sun

Do you have the courage to go a bit deeper? Let's consider the analogy of an avocado and the sun. Your heart and emotions are intricately woven together. Here, I'm talking about your whole heart, your physical and energetic heart. Think of your emotions and heart as an avocado and the sun. The avocado has an outer hard shell—like what you show people on the outside. That's what people see when they see you, and it tends to be their first impression of you. You might think of your shell as how you are trying to appear to others, even if it doesn't align with how you feel inside. For example, trying to come off as confident but not feeling it, or smiling or acting calm when feeling anxious. Or acting tough when you're as tenderhearted as a teddy bear. Your shell is also part of your shield.

Underneath the shell of the avocado is the soft part: there's so much going on underneath the surface in every one of us that is not immediately noticeable to most people. There are a lot of these squishy feelings underneath, and you may or may not be in touch with yourself. This can also feel confusing. We'll discuss how to deal with those emotions in just a moment. For now, let's continue to look at the analogy of the different layers in an avocado.

In the middle of the avocado is the pit, or the core, representing your core emotions. It's also the core of how these emotions came to be, your core patterns. A lot of this tends to be subconscious. Grief and sadness are often at the core. But there may be so much covering up the core emotions that on the outside (the shell), a person can look like they're doing okay, and in a way, they might be, but people don't see what's going on underneath the surface. There are so many stories of people feeling depressed, and friends and family saying they never knew.

The various emotions can be at any layer. For example, maybe there's a hidden guilt on the inside. When a loved one passes, for instance, it's common to feel guilty over things that happened, but that guilt is a cover for the core emotion of sadness. Sometimes, the anger or shame people feel can be hidden in the soft part—again, those emotions tend to be a cover for sadness.

Remember, there's nothing wrong with the hard shell or the soft part covering the core. Those middle and outer layers are there because core emotions often feel overwhelming. It's good to have coping mechanisms when things are overwhelming because they get us through. There's no judgment here on what we're feeling.

Deep down, past the shell, the flesh, and the core emotions, is the sun—this is the light of your soul. It never goes out. It is everlasting and shines even beneath the many other layers. That sun is your heart center. It's difficult to feel when the heart is aching. Remember, though, the reason you hurt is because you love. You love yourself. You love another being. You love the earth. When you realize this, you see the deeper meaning behind your hurt, and this understanding brings a kind of joyfulness even to the grief you feel. As your self-understanding grows and you can see the layers of yourself, the various emotions are processed and lightened. The core emotions no longer eclipse the sun. You become transparent to yourself, which means you can see the sun's light within you.

Figure 2 - The Avocado and the Sun: Emotional "Layers"

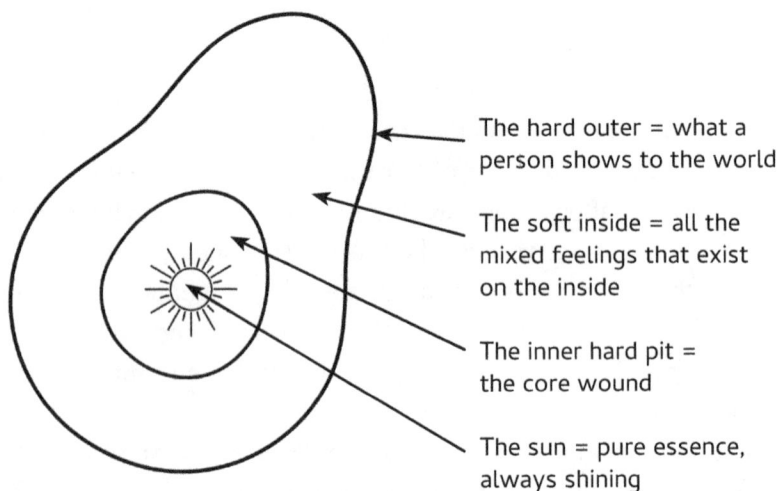

The hard outer = what a person shows to the world

The soft inside = all the mixed feelings that exist on the inside

The inner hard pit = the core wound

The sun = pure essence, always shining

Next, let's make this analogy of the avocado and the sun more practical. You might be wondering how to approach your emotional layers and how to access the light and love of your heart, especially when you are hurting. Keep reading.

A Four-Step Process for Difficult Emotions

How do you approach difficult emotions? With so many layers, it can feel like you might unravel if you lift one. So, it takes courage to see beyond these layers and acknowledge the difficult emotions there. We approach those tender feelings gently, as we would a baby. When a baby fusses, we embrace and softly hug the baby. We don't demand the baby stop crying (it wouldn't work anyway). It's the same with a scared animal. We have to have so much patience, or else it might lash out or run away and hide. So you can't rush the process. You love, love, love. And in that love nest, the baby is soothed in time. That's how you can approach your tender spots, too. Cradle the anger, sadness, frustration, grief, and any uncomfortable emotion with love, as you would a baby.

Using that gentle approach, here's a four-step process to help you through difficult emotions. This step-by-step process will help you put down your heart shield and open your heart. Understanding the process also helps satisfy both the right and left sides of your brain (the masculine and feminine aspects), enabling you to access more of your abilities.

You can use this process anywhere, anytime. If you're new to this kind of self-awareness practice, then take care to find a quiet, safe space that is relatively free from distractions. How long you spend doing the practice can vary depending on what feels helpful for you. You could go through it in minutes, an hour, or longer. You could even use this four-step process in the spur of the moment. There are no hard rules when doing this. See what works for you at different times, and get professional help if needed.

Step 1: Ask yourself what you are feeling.

Take a moment to notice your emotions without any judgment. What do you feel? Just name each of the emotions you're feeling: I feel sad, I feel angry, I feel frustrated, etc. If you need help finding words to describe your feelings, use the Vocabulary of Emotions table I've included here. Chances are you are experiencing multiple emotions. You can also experience opposite emotions simultaneously, such as

Table 6 - A Vocabulary of Emotions

LOVE

Joy

Adorable
Adventurous
Affectionate
Alert
Amazed
Amused
Appreciated
Assured
Astounded
Awed
Beaming
Beautiful
Blissful
Bold
Bright
Buoyant
Capable
Caring
Celebratory
Certain
Charmed
Cheeky
Cheerful
Cherished
Childish
Chipper
Clever
Comical
Compassionate
Connected
Creative
Curious
Daring
Dear
Delighted
Desirable
Determined
Eager
Ecstatic
Elated
Electrified
Empowered
Enamored
Enchanted
Endearing
Energetic
Engaged
Enraptured
Enthusiastic

Euphoric
Expansive
Expectant
Exploring
Expressive
Exuberant
Fascinated
Festive
Flirtatious
Free
Full
Fun
Funny
Gay
Glad
Good
Good-humored
Groovy
Happy
Happy-go-lucky
Healthy
Heartwarming
Heavenly
Helpful
High
Honored
Hopeful
Incredible
Infatuated
Intimate
Inspired
Inquisitive
Intrigued
Invigorated
Jolly
Joyful
Kind
Lighthearted
Loving
Magnificent
Merry
Motivated
Optimistic
Over-the-moon
Passionate
Peppy
Playful
Positive
Pretty
Proud
Radiant
Renewed
Resplendent

Respected
Romantic
Satisfied
Sexy
Silly
Smiley
Sparkling
Successful
Sunny
Talkative
Tender-hearted
Thrilled
Upbeat
Valued
Vibrant
Vivacious
Warm-hearted
Wonderful
Zany

Gratitude

Appreciative
Blessed
Fortunate
Generous
Glad
Grateful
Gratifying
Humbled
Moved
Relieved
Thankful
Thoughtful

Peace

Accepting
Adequate
Amiable
Angelic
At Ease
Benevolent
Brave
Breezy
Calm
Carefree
Centered
Comforted
Considerate
Connected
Content
Courageous

Eternal
Forgiven
Fortunate
Friendly
Fulfilled
Gentle
Graceful
Grounded
Hopeful
Infinite
Limitless
Lucky
Meditative
Mindful
Pleasant
Prepared
Present
Refreshed
Relaxed
Reverent
Serene
Safe
Trusting
Warm
Welcome
Worthy

FEAR

Anger

Aggravated
Aggressive
Angry
Annoyed
Argumentative
Bad
Burned Out
Contempt
Cold
Combative
Cool
Cranky
Crazy
Critical
Cursed
Cynical
Deceitful
Destructive
Disapproving
Disdainful
Disgruntled
Dismayed

Dismissive	Agony	Hated	Screwed Up
Dissatisfied	Aloof	Heartbroken	Shameful
Distant	Anguished	Helpless	Shut Down
Envious	Anxious	Hesitant	Shy
Evil	Apathetic	Homesick	Sick
Exasperated	Ashamed	Hopeless	Sorrowful
Forced	Awful	Horrible	Tearful
Frustrated	Bitter	Hurt	Terrible
Furious	Blah	Hysterical	Terrified
Grouchy	Blue	Ignored	Thwarted
Hostile	Burdened	Imposed Upon	Tragic
Impatient	Cheated	Inconsolable	Trapped
Irritated	Concerned	Inadequate	Troubled
Jealous	Condemned	Indifferent	Ugly
Judgmental	Crestfallen	Inferior	Uneasy
Hateful	Crushed	Inhibited	Unenthusiastic
Hostile	Defeated	Insecure	Unfeeling
Humiliated	Depressed	Insignificant	Unfortunate
Indignant	Despised	Isolated	Unhappy
Infuriated	Despair	Jaded	Unimportant
Irate	Diminished	Judged	Unsettled
Irritated	Disabled	Jumpy	Unsure
Lecherous	Disappointed	Left Out	Victimized
Loathing	Discouraged	Listless	Vulnerable
Let Down	Dismal	Lonely	Weak
Mad	Disoriented	Longing	Weary
Mean	Despondent	Low	Weepy
Mistrustful	Distressed	Melancholy	Withdrawn
Moody	Disturbed	Miserable	Woeful
Numb	Doleful	Mortified	Worn Out
Obnoxious	Dominated	Mournful	Worried
Out of Control	Doubtful	Neglected	Worthless
Outraged	Down	Offended	Wretched
Quarrelsome	Downcast	Old	Yearning
Pissed	Downhearted	Out of sorts	
Provoked	Drained	Overwhelmed	**Disgust**
Ridiculed	Dull	Panicked	
Rushed	Edgy	Paralyzed	Repelled
Shocked	Embarrassed	Pathetic	Repulsed
Sneaky	Excluded	Persecuted	Revolted
Spiteful	Exhausted	Petrified	
Stingy	Foolish	Pressured	**Other**
Suspicious	Forgotten	Rattled	
Threatened	Forlorn	Regretful	Bored
Upset	Fragile	Reluctant	Confused
Vengeful	Frantic	Remorseful	Hungry
Vindictive	Frazzled	Rejected	Questioning
Violated	Frightened	Resigned	Perplexed
	Gloomy	Self-conscious	Sensitive
Grief	Glum	Silenced	Shy
	Grief-stricken	Startled	Sleepy
Abandoned	Guilty	Sad	Thirsty
Afraid	Gullible	Scared	

joyful grief. This range makes for the whole human experience. So, name all the aspects of your feelings, including those that don't seem to make sense. Calling out how you feel helps you to be present with your experience and helps to keep you grounded. You are allowing yourself to feel whatever you feel, and being able to witness yourself, no matter what you are going through, is loving yourself.

Step 2: Where do you feel that in your body?

Next, ask yourself where in the body you feel the emotions. Is there tension in the head, neck, and shoulders? Pressure in the chest? Butterflies or a pit in the belly? A numbness or tingling sensation anywhere? Whatever physical sensations you feel, call those out. If you need more words to describe the sensations in your body, use the following table. And again, be a neutral and loving witness to yourself and your experience; allow yourself to feel your body.

Table 7 - A Vocabulary of Body Sensations

Achy	Expanded	Pounding	Squeezing
Airy	Faint	Pressure	Sticky
Alive	Fatigued	Prickly	Stiff
Blocked	Floating	Puffy	Still
Breathless	Flowing	Pulled	Stinging
Bruised	Fluid	Pulsating	Streaming
Bubbly	Flushed	Quaking	Stretchy
Burning	Fluttery	Queasy	Stringy
Buzzing	Frozen	Quiet	Strong
Calm	Full	Quivering	Suffocating
Clammy	Fuzzy	Radiating	Sweaty
Chilled	Hard	Ragged	Tender
Clenched	Heavy	Raw	Tense
Closed	Hollow	Relaxed	Thick
Congested	Hot	Releasing	Tickling
Constricted	Icy	Rolling	Tight
Contracted	Intense	Sensitive	Tingling
Cold	Itchy	Settled	Tired
Cool	Jumpy	Shaky	Trembling
Cozy	Knotted	Sharp	Twitchy
Crawling	Light	Shivery	Vibrating
Dark	Limp	Silky	Warm
Dense	Loose	Smooth	Weak
Dizzy	Magical	Soft	Weight on chest
Drained	Nauseated	Sore	Weight on
Dull	Numb	Spacey	shoulders
Electric	Open	Spacious	Wobbly
Empty	Painful	Sparkly	Wooden
Energized	Paralyzed	Spasming	

Step 3: Are you breathing?

Next, check on your breathing. How are you breathing? Are you breathing? Ever so gently, introduce some movement into your breath. Just ease it in. Let your breath move into the tense areas of your body and the emotions you feel. Your breath will give you the necessary momentum to help you process your experience.

Step 4: Feel the sun.

This is a bonus step. I don't always include it, but I didn't want to leave it out here because it can be key to healing. Inside you, your true self is light and love. If you can feel this, that love can radiate all around you and encompass any experience you've had, are having, and will have. (We'll keep unpacking this truth throughout the book.)

An alternate way to do this four-step process is to switch steps 1 and 2. Start with what you feel in your body, and then inquire where you feel this way in your life. Doing it in this order can be helpful for more analytical types who have trouble identifying their emotions.

I've walked myself through these steps many times in my life, including during tragic times, which I say more about in chapter 8. However, I also like to do this practice throughout the day whenever I feel triggered. That way, I help myself process emotions immediately instead of storing them away for another time. I'll also do an abbreviated version in seconds at the start of any difficult encounter and check in with myself again afterward.

For example, I had a patient I'll call Frank come into my office, but he was not happy about being there. His wife had scheduled his appointment with me. Frank directed his anger at me and said he didn't know why he was there and didn't think I could help him because he had tried everything. Initially, I was taken aback by his aggressive demeanor. Physically, I'm a little person, and when someone larger than you speaks to you in an angry way, it can be intimidating. I had to ground myself quickly to respond to the situation in the best way possible.

I walked myself through the four steps:

1. What was I feeling? I felt afraid of someone directing their booming voice and anger at me. (It's okay to feel afraid.)

2. What was I feeling in my body? I felt my shoulders tense up. (It's okay to feel this way.)

3. Was I breathing? Not completely. So I started moving my breath, slow and steady, which helped me ground my fear and relaxed my shoulders.

4. Feel the sun. Because I could feel my self-love, it was easier for me to respond more lovingly rather than defensively.

   And then I spoke to Frank. "I understand that you are angry and frustrated with your situation and that you say you've tried everything," I told him. "You also said you don't like being angry and didn't used to be this way. As you know, emotions can affect our health, so if you haven't addressed your anger, I suggest we start there."

In moments like this one with Frank, my love for myself motivates me to go through this four-step process. I know that feeling is healing, so I'm willing to take the steps to heal. Getting here has taken me years of practice, but it doesn't have to take you that long. Use the exercises in this book. Regularly and earnestly. Taking the time to get to know and understand yourself, to dig deeper, is always worthwhile. And you are worth it.

Summary

In this chapter, you learned what grounding is and what keeps you from being grounded. When we ground, we let built-up energy discharge into the ground—in the same way that an electrical circuit needs to be grounded for stability to prevent electrical shock.

- Grounding helps to stabilize your energy field.

- You can determine whether or not you are grounded based on signs from your body, emotions, mind, and spirit. Being grounded feels more balanced and steady.

- Many factors can make it difficult to ground, including these:
  - An unbalanced and nutrient-deprived diet
  - Chaotic energy in the environment
  - Spending too much time indoors
  - Generational trauma
  - Resisting emotional challenges

- When you feel the need to protect your heart, it's common to put up a protective heart shield, which has both physical and energetic aspects. The heart shield creates more heaviness in the body and can prevent you from fully living.

- Gathering the courage to be vulnerable and lower your heart shield will help you ground.

- Mindful movement helps you process "e-motions."

- Understanding various breathing patterns will give you insight into yourself and how to use your breath to ground.

- You and your emotions are like an avocado, with a hard outer shell, a soft inside, and core emotions at the pit. At the center of the pit is the shining light of your heart center, which is ever-present no matter what might be covering it.

- Feeling is healing. You can use the four-step process to go deeper.

- When we are more grounded and present in the body, we're more prepared to listen to the body's intuition. In the next chapter, we dive deeper into how to read the body's compass.

CHAPTER 3

READING YOUR BODY'S COMPASS

"Learning to use the body's compass takes courage
and a desire to know yourself fully."

When I was in my mid-twenties, I had a hunch that if I didn't make a major change in how I was living, I was going to get sick. The doctors said I was fine. Nothing was wrong with me aside from some minor reflux that kept me up at night. I was given antacids to take care of that, a simple solution, yet something in my body didn't sit right.

Walking to the post office one day, I noticed a yoga sign. Something in my gut told me to walk in. Within a few weeks of taking yoga classes, my reflux disappeared without antacids and never returned. I also felt more centered while working in the emergency room, even during a crisis. A couple of staff members even commented on the change.

I'm so glad I decided to listen to my body's message to make a change. By listening to my body, I made the crucial decision to pivot my life. My body's compass sent me in a new direction, one in which I felt more comfortable with myself and could follow my truth. In this chapter, I've put together some key concepts to help you tap into your body's intuition and compass.

Know Your Constitution

In the holistic world, you'll get used to more fluid qualities. Being sensitive, for example, is a gradient, just as being grounded is. It's not all or nothing. At one end, someone with a highly sensitive constitution functions more like a sports car. If they are a little off balance, they can *feel* way off because they notice even minor changes easily. Fortunately, a little fine-tuning can also go a long way for such people. At the other end of the gradient, someone with a less sensitive constitution handles more like a Mack truck. They appear strong and hearty, and it takes a lot to throw them off course. But when they get into trouble, they can be thrown way off course, and it might take more to get them back on track. Of course, these are generalities; there can be any variation. The degree of sensitivity may not be the same in every dimension of a person's body, mind, and spirit, and where we are on these gradients can change as we grow and evolve.

People with more sensitive physical constitutions are more likely to react to medications and supplements, perhaps needing lower doses. As a pediatrician, I know that pediatricians adjust medication doses according to the child's weight. But while there's at least some individualization in pediatric medicine, it is not yet commonplace to consider an adult's constitution for all medication dosing. Oddly, in adult medicine, there tends to be one dosage, regardless of a person's size or constitution. This means a petite 110-pound woman will be given the same dosage as a 300-pound man. In geriatric medicine, physicians again consider smaller dosages because there is some understanding that older adults may be more sensitive to medications than younger adults. There is currently a trend toward personalized medicine, where the art of medicine comes into play, which I'll discuss more in chapter 11.

Many of my patients tend to have sensitive constitutions. Taking note of a person's constitution is one of the first things I do as an integrative physician. For everyone, it's important to listen to your body when starting any new regimen, whether a new exercise, diet, supplement, or medication. A rule of thumb is to start low and slow, then make small, incremental adjustments as needed. Titrating doses gives time for the body to adjust and get used to the "new" thing. More is not necessarily better—for example, if you're dehydrated, you don't need gallons of water. Titrating also allows time to notice reactions and determine the ideal dose. I'm fairly sensitive to herbs. There's a common tea with senna that's used for constipation. The adult recommendation is one cup. I can drink only a quarter of a cup. More than that, and my belly starts cramping. Have you ever overdone it? There's not a one-size-fits-all. We're all unique. So, make no assumptions and follow the rule of thumb to start low and slow.

Some people are also more sensitive to the vibrations around them. Have you ever walked into a building and felt it had a strange vibe or walked into a home that felt warm and welcoming? You could be picking up on the energy of the space, the people in the area, or even the electromagnetic fields. Most people can sense some energy. They might also be able to describe it if they place their awareness on it. Some people tend to feel things physically more than others; they have a visceral reaction. They are described as highly sensitive or empathic. In general, kids tend to be more sensitive to energy than adults.

Whether you're a born empath or learn to strengthen your sensitivities, these abilities are a gift—though they may not always feel that way because sensitivity brings a host of issues. You could feel overwhelmed and pushed around by your senses as if lost at sea, or you might have difficulty focusing and feeling clear. However, if you learn how to sense things from a more neutral perspective, your sensitivities will make you very good at picking up details, which can be helpful in anything you do. Your keen senses will give you more data points to inform and guide your decisions. The more you understand about yourself, the easier it is to know what steps to take for further healing and growth. This leads us to another question: How do you know if what you are feeling is coming from you or what's around you?

Deciphering Another's Emotions from Your Own

It can sometimes be difficult for empaths to maintain their identity and sense of self because they take in so much sensory input from the world that their emotions can feel like a jumble of confusion. Empaths feel what other people feel. If you can't distinguish your energy from the energy of others, you risk taking on others' emotions. It doesn't feel great to soak up the feelings around you constantly. At any given moment, a lot is going on in the world, and if you keep absorbing like a sponge, without discernment, you could end up in a constant state of anxiety.

Have you ever interacted with someone and it felt awkward, but you weren't sure why? You only know that the person's expression, words, and actions didn't line up with what you felt from them. For example, a teacher or a co-worker might have had a rough weekend and feel pretty stressed by Monday. Although they try to do their job and act professionally, covering up what they feel inside, the empathic person will pick up on incongruent nuances. Hence, the awkward feelings. What you need to do in such a situation is pause, back up, and consider what you're sensing as neutral data points. In our example, those neutral data points might be:

- Something feels awkward.

- My co-worker is smiling, but her words don't feel happy.

- Her forehead looks tense.

Do you see the incongruencies? She is smiling, but there's tension in her face and words. That's why you sense awkwardness.

There are many possible explanations for why things don't line up, but you don't have to figure them all out. What's essential for your clarity is understanding that you are picking up on vibrations around you; then, choose to observe what is coming in without taking it on as yours.

When you sponge up the emotional vibrations of others, it feels like static in your energy field (I'll say more about static in your energy field later in this chapter). An Energy Field Massage can be a helpful first step to gain some clarity. You simply use your hands to gently massage and loosen up the static in your energy field. To do this, first wake up the energy points on your hands by rubbing your palms together briskly, as you would to warm up your hands. Bring your awareness to your hands as they warm up to heighten the sensing abilities of your hands; your palms act like another set of eyes or antennas.

Next, use your hands to gently comb through your energy field, which extends about six to twelve inches off your physical body. Move your hands to smooth out your energy field from top to bottom. You're giving yourself a subtle energy massage and brushing off the static in your field. You might notice little ripples, spikes, or tangles in some areas more than others. These represent static in your field. No need to be alarmed—simply smooth these out with your palms. You can also shake your hands toward the earth to ground the excess charge. Imagine shaking your hands into a compost pile where the excess charge can transform into something nourishing. You could also stomp your feet to help ground that extra static charge. See how you feel after a few minutes of this subtle energy massage. Detangling Your Cords on page 82 is a good follow-up exercise to this one.

The more grounded you are, the easier it is to observe and not take on what isn't yours. Then, you'll be able to listen to your body's messages, which will make a big difference in your life. At this point, you may question how to recognize when you should listen to fear and when to persist despite fear. We will cover this later in this chapter. For now, let's finish laying the foundation that will help you better understand your body's compass.

What Kind of Intuitive Are You?

Do you know that you are intuitive? It's true, even if you're not aware of it. Although some constitutions are naturally more intuitive than others, intuition is an ability anyone can cultivate. It's like the ability to sing. Anyone can sing, but some people can naturally sing better than others. Whether or not you're a born singer, if you practice, you will develop your singing abilities to be better than they were. The same goes for intuition: you can learn to develop your intuitive abilities. This book will help you develop your intuition and fine-tune the intuitive gift you may already use.

Read the following statements and check the boxes next to the ones that ring true for you. This will give you a better sense of the kind of intuition you have.

Intuitive Feeling

☐ I cry easily at movies.

☐ When other people are in pain, I feel their discomfort in my body.

☐ I don't feel comfortable buying vintage or used clothing.

☐ When I walk into a crowd, I easily feel overwhelmed.

☐ I can read the energy in a room as soon as I walk in.

Intuitive Seeing

☐ Sometimes, I have premonitions or dreams that come true.

☐ I can see images in my mind when someone tells me a story.

☐ When something catches my eye, I know it's for a reason.

☐ I dress in colors that match my mood.

☐ I am drawn to abstract paintings.

Intuitive Hearing

☐ Music has a strong impact on my emotions.

☐ I'm sensitive to sound and the volume of different sounds. I don't like loud sounds.

☐ I seek out quiet when I am overwhelmed.

☐ I seek out soothing music for calm.

☐ I can hear whispers of guidance from within myself.

Intuitive Smelling

☐ I can enter a room and tell if something "smells off."

☐ I sometimes smell things that are not in my immediate surroundings.

☐ I can smell the presence of a loved one who has crossed over.

☐ I can smell whether someone is telling the truth.

☐ Smells can bring back strong memories.

Intuitive Knowing

☐ I can tell when people are insincere or lying, even when others can't.

☐ I easily confuse other people's thoughts with my own, especially when I'm not grounded.

☐ I often think about a person just before they call or message me.

☐ Sometimes, I know things without knowing how I know them.

☐ Sometimes, I experience déjà vu.

Channeling (direct communication with spirit)

☐ I feel the presence of angels, guides, or loved ones who have crossed over.

☐ I see or have seen angels or spirits.

☐ I can see or have seen a glow or an aura around people.

☐ Loved ones who have crossed over give me messages in my dreams.

☐ I have conversations with loved ones who have crossed over.

The more boxes you check, the more sensitive or naturally intuitive you are. Did you check off more boxes in specific categories? This lets you know which extrasensory skills you might be more inclined to develop. If you didn't check off any of the boxes, that doesn't mean you aren't intuitive. Practice and grounding can help anyone open up their self-awareness and intuition. The exercises in this book will help you do this.

Here's more information on each category of intuitive abilities:

- **Intuitive Feeling, aka clairsentience (clear feeling)—the feeler**
This is the most common type of intuition for empaths. You feel, and your body has a visceral response to the things you pick up on. People might have told you you're too sensitive. You might be picky about where you stand in a room or sit at a restaurant. Keep developing this mind-body connection as you learn to discern what your intuition is telling you without getting overwhelmed.

- **Intuitive Seeing, aka clairvoyance (clear seeing)—the seer**
You're a visual person who can easily imagine and dream. Color is important in your life. You might let your imagination get the best of you and run you down. Keep developing a gentle awareness of your visual abilities so that you can tap into your gifts as a visionary and uplift your life and the lives of others.

- **Intuitive Hearing, aka clairaudience (clear hearing)—the telepath**
  Sound can be your friend or foe. Your ears might ring now and then when your guides want to get your attention. Be patient with yourself as you learn to listen to whatever messages come through. It's okay to have periods of silence to listen to your inner guidance. It's also okay to surround yourself with healing music.

- **Intuitive Smelling, aka clairolfactance or clairsalience (clear smelling)—the nose that knows**
  Do not underestimate this lesser-known intuitive ability. The olfactory bulb directly connects to the brain and is part of the limbic system, which is important in memory and emotions. You tend to be good at picking up scents and sniffing out people, places, things, and situations. You might be put off by odors even when others aren't. Intuitive smell is closely related to intuitive taste since about 80 percent of our sense of taste is connected to smell.

- **Intuitive Knowing, aka claircognizance (clear knowing)—the sage**
  You've got some good wits and hunches. You can read people pretty easily. You can read interactions between people in a way that is not apparent to others. You do this so easily that you might take offense when people do not respond as you think they should. Keep getting to know yourself and your constitution so that you better understand that the way other people behave is not personal, even though it can feel like it.

- **Channeling—the prophet**
  Chances are you've experienced a variety of intuitive happenings through multiple intuitive senses. Some people are so clear that the information comes through them more directly. It's okay to be different, but don't expect everyone to know what you know. Be gentle with yourself as you learn to manage and fine-tune your abilities.

These categories are not meant to define you as a feeler, seer, telepath, sage, or prophet. The terms are not a certification, nor do they imply any mastery. Instead, they are descriptive and fluid and meant to help you realize the potential of your abilities. It takes practice to understand your sensitivities and intuitive potential. Recognizing the patterns you pick up on can help you gain an overall understanding.

Next, let's go through the general patterns commonly observed in a person's subtle energy field.

Reading Your Subtle Energy Body

Your subtle energy body is the rainbow body of light around you that is not visible to the regular eye unless you have extrasensory abilities. The subtle energy body has many other names, including the light body, the rainbow body, the energy field, the biofield, or the aura. Although there are nuances to these terms, don't get too bogged down in the wording. There are also many details and dimensions to the subtle energy body. Let's focus on the gestalt (the organized whole, which is perceived as more than the sum of its parts.)

Over the years, I've noticed in my patients various patterns in the shapes and locations of the subtle energy body in relationship to the physical body. Here's a table of the simple patterns I see and what they could represent. In reality, the shape of your energy body can be any combination of these patterns, so there are infinite shapes that your energy body could manifest. The shape of your energy body is also fluid, not static; it is an expression of your living being. Despite the ever-changing nature of your energy field, I find this simple table helpful, as there can be a general pattern that your energy field expresses more than others.

Aligned and symmetric: A healthy energy field surrounds the body in a balanced way. The body, mind, and spirit are fully aligned. The person is grounded in their body and fully present in the moment. To help you maintain a balanced field, regularly practice the Opening and Centering Your Heart Field exercise on page 81. This is also a great exercise to address imbalances in the energy field; it helps open spiky, curled-in, or shrunken energy fields and centers the field with your heart and physical body.

Spiky shape: If the subtle energy body has spikes in its shape, there is some static and confusion in the person's field. The subtle energy body is not as clear and smooth as it could be. The person could have diffi-

Table 8 - The Shape and Location of Your Energy Field

Location or shape of the subtle energy body in relationship to the physical body	Possible meaning
Aligned and symmetric	Balanced energy field
Spiky shape	Static in the energy field, some confusion, difficulty letting go of certain things
Head curled into the heart	Heart shield, hiding like an ostrich with its head in the sand
Behind	Hiding behind yourself (flight)
In front	On guard and hyperalert, often with tunnel vision (fight)
Partially above	Ungrounded
Completely above	Dissociated
To the right	Masculine emphasis, ignoring the feminine side
To the left	Feminine emphasis, ignoring the masculine side
Shrunken field	A crushed heart, shielding, retreating inward to disconnect, like a turtle pulled into its shell
Without boundaries	No container, too open, easily overwhelmed, difficulty distinguishing self from others and the environment

culty letting go of certain things, including looping thoughts and emotions. The confusion in the field can also be from sponging up others' emotions. The Energy Field Massage described earlier helps smooth out static and confusion in your field.

Head curled into the heart: Like an ostrich with its head in the sand, this is a protective mechanism that creates a heart shield. Recall from chapter 2 that although it's common to have a heart shield, it does keep emotions stuck and ungrounds your energy field. See the Lowering Your Heart Shield exercise on page 37, as well as Opening Up Your Wings on page 38.

Behind: When the subtle energy body is located behind the physical body, you are hiding behind yourself, stuck in a flight response, and not fully sharing your gifts with the world. This is common in sensitive people who may be shy or hesitant. This was me for so long. I wanted to blend in even when I was different. Part of me was content being a snail hiding in my shell, but I was keeping myself from my full potential. It's taken me years into adulthood to be more comfortable outside my shell. Simple breathing exercises, such as the Long Exhale on page 42, can be helpful to calm the nervous system.

In front: When the subtle energy body is located in front of the physical body, you could be hyperalert and on guard, a bit stuck in that fight response. You keep people at arm's length; they never get to know the true you. It can be hard to develop intimate relationships this way. You prefer to shield yourself from harm rather than expose any vulnerability. I've been there too. Again, the breathing exercises in chapter 2, such as The Space Between on page 43, can be helpful here.

Partially above: Many people walk around with their subtle energy bodies partially above them. When we overthink, we become "heady" and ungrounded. Feeling into your feet is harder when you're partly ungrounded because you're partly dissociated from your body. Take note of whether you can feel the upper half of your body the same as the lower half. These days, with computer and phone use and working at desks, it's easy to become ungrounded in this way. Go back to chapter 2 to find the grounding exercises there. Progressive Muscle Relaxation, an exercise on page 79 can also help.

Completely above: When the subtle energy body is completely above the physical body, you are probably unaware of it because you've disassociated. You could feel like you're "out of your body." Numbing out is not a sustainable way to live. If you're not present in your life, your body becomes a machine running stuck patterns rather than the home

of a conscious being, which it's meant to be. You are not fully dissociated if you understand what you're reading in this book. It's a gradient,
so it's possible to be partially dissociated or ungrounded. If you feel
yourself starting to dissociate or flood, bring awareness to the lower
half of your body and stomp your feet. Also, do the Five Senses Meditation for Grounding described on page 78. If you feel flooded and
numbed out frequently, consider getting professional help.

To the right: The right side of the body is more masculine, so if the subtle energy body preferentially stays on this side, you are ignoring your
left side or energetically feminine side. Chances are that raw, unprocessed emotions have been tucked away and ignored. This can happen
whether you are biologically male or female. I first noticed this when a
businessman I'll call Tom came to see me. I was a bit perplexed by the
stark contrast in the location of his physical and energetic bodies. Fortunately, I was able to talk candidly to him about it. I mentioned that
there might be unprocessed emotions for him to address. His response
made total sense: "I try to crush out any emotion," he told me. No
wonder his energy body was like that! When the subtle energy body
shifts to the right, it also means there are untapped feminine strengths
for the person to access—maybe being more creative or perhaps rebalancing relationships with feminine figures. The exercises on pages 22
and 75 involving cross-lateral movements and integrating the left and
right sides will help with the needed rebalancing.

To the left: When the subtle energy body is to the left of the physical body, you prefer energetically feminine thoughts and expression.
You are comfortable talking about emotions, though you may still
have a hard time balancing life because we need both our masculine
and feminine energies to live fully in this world. When I see people in
this energetic state, they might need to work on practical matters such
as their schedules, finances, or any other business requiring logistics
and planning. No matter how enlightened we are, there are still bills
and taxes! Planning could also be about scheduling time for self-care.
With this imbalance, relationships with male figures in your life may
need balancing. Anytime there is a right-left imbalance, it helps to

incorporate cross-lateral movements. As noted above, the cross-lateral exercises on pages 22 and 75 will be helpful here.

Shrunken field: Here, the subtle energy body is pulled in and contracted, allowing you to retreat into yourself. This is a way to disconnect from the world. You don't feel interested in engaging in the world. Your energy and mood may feel down. Perhaps you were hurt in the past, and this is how you learned to cope. There's very little momentum in this state. That you're reading this book is a good sign. Every little step you take will create some movement. Being in nature will also be helpful—being in nature is beneficial for any unbalanced energy state.

Without boundaries: There is such a thing as being too open. Even your energy field needs a boundary or container (we will discuss boundaries further in part 2). When your energy field is too wide open, you will have difficulty distinguishing yourself from others. Yes, I know we are part of the Oneness of all life, but for this human existence, we must also understand who we are as individuals; otherwise, it can feel like the deep ocean waves have swept us away. When your field is wide open, you will easily be overwhelmed by the thoughts, emotions, and energies around you. There can be a tendency to dissociate, making it important to get professional help from a medical or mental health practitioner.

Try this Sphere of Stardust exercise to help you create a clear boundary for your energy field. *Imagine yourself in a giant sphere. Let that sphere fill with stardust so that your whole body, energy field, and the environment around you are encompassed. Give yourself a moment to feel and breathe in this light. Then, within this sphere, imagine an egg-shaped field around you representing your energy field. Let that egg-shaped field sparkle with any color or colors you choose, and imagine the colors within the egg-shaped field freely expressing themselves. The sphere of stardust continues to surround and permeate the egg-shaped field like a comforting and protective nest. Know that you are always loved and protected; your egg-shaped field can express freely within this nourishing nest of light.*

There are ways to perceive the subtle energy body with your feeling-knowing intuition, where you feel your energy field in relation to your body or someone else's in relation to theirs. This could feel like more presence in some areas than others. If you were to scan your whole body with your awareness, you might feel a particular area of the body is easier to notice than others, or it could feel like a projection of another person's energy is shifted in one direction or another compared to their physical body. Are you living in the center of your rainbow, or is it off-kilter? To strengthen your perception and care for the subtle energy body, practice the exercises in Part 1 called Massaging Your Energy Field and Your Rainbow Body on page 84.

Revisiting the Body's Symptoms and Messages

As we discussed in chapter 1, your body's symptoms are its way of communicating with you. The amazing thing is that they also point to where the healing is. The symptoms show us what to tend to both physically and metaphorically. So, there's no need to be afraid of your symptoms. Instead of fighting them, listen to them. Lean into your symptoms; breathe into them to help you listen. What message is coming through?

Let's go through the example of adrenal fatigue, which most people experience at some point in their lives. Your adrenal glands make stress hormones and hormones that help balance your salt levels, sugar levels, blood pressure, and sex hormones. When you are faced with intense or prolonged stress, your adrenal glands might be unable to keep up with the production of hormones needed to respond to the stress. When that happens, it is called "adrenal fatigue" or "adrenal insufficiency." (In medical terms, adrenal fatigue is also known as HPA-axis dysfunction. "H" is for the hypothalamus, "P" is for the pituitary, and "A" is for the adrenals. The hypothalamus sends messages to the pituitary, which sends messages to the adrenals. Then there's a feedback loop from the adrenals back to the hypothalamus and pituitary.)

Signs of adrenal fatigue include fatigue, anxiety; irritability; insomnia; low libido; weight gain, especially around the abdominal area; blood pressure imbalances; hypoglycemic symptoms; and salt, sugar, and caffeine cravings. Symptoms can range from mild to severe depending on how tired the adrenals are.

As soon as your body starts to reach its limits, it sends a message to let you know some changes are needed. The messages are subtle at first, as simple as feeling tired. You could ignore the feeling and power through with sugar and caffeine instead of slowing down and resting. But as the adrenal fatigue worsens, it will be harder to ignore the signs. You'll start to feel both wired and tired—your engine is now sputtering. You could feel tired all day but then have a second wind and be wide awake at night. The body's rhythms are out of sorts, pleading with you: "I'm really tired! Please do something!" or "Please stop doing so many things!" If you keep ignoring these symptoms, eventually the adrenals will run out of steam, and you'll feel tired all the time, from the moment you wake up until night. At this point, your body has taken over. It is no longer waiting for you to make a change; it is making you change. Now you have no choice but to rest because you don't have the energy to get through the day. You must slow down, rest, and replenish yourself.

Do you see how the body's messages are trying to help you? In the case of adrenal fatigue, the symptom of fatigue is not bad. It doesn't feel good, but that doesn't mean your body is working against you. Typically, it's the other way around, where we work against our bodies. Let your analytical mind consider the symptoms as data points that are trying to guide you towards balance.

When you use your intuition to tune in to your body, you can pick up on its signals sooner. For example, you could tune in to your body's energy field to get an overview of your emotional body. With adrenal fatigue, you could look at the energetic properties of the organ systems we discussed in chapter 1. The adrenals sit on top of the kidneys. They are closely related to the kidneys' energetic properties, which include fear, grief, and sadness—tender emotions that need processing. (Chapter 2 and the exercises at the end of Part I provide help with this.) Intuiting the body's symptoms is about feeling into healing. The sooner you listen to your body, the easier the healing steps. But if you wait until later, more drastic changes may be required. So, prioritize your self-care one step at a time.

When to Listen to Fear

When should we listen to fear, and when should we persist despite it? Well, partly that depends on our goals. Is the fear keeping you from taking a step toward your dreams? Then, chances are the fear is your ego mind trying to keep you in the box it knows (more on ego later in the book). In this case, you need to keep going. Or, is the fear redirecting you, like a flash of intuition, asking you to switch gears or change perspective, maybe even a 180-degree turnaround?

One way to determine whether to ignore your fear (ego) or listen to it (intuition) is to use your body as a compass and ask it questions. Your body subconsciously takes in information, especially through the solar plexus. Have you ever heard of a "gut instinct?" This is what's at play. Your body is continually receiving information and giving you feedback, and it responds faster than your thoughts can process.

Ways to Access Your Body's Wisdom

Use your body as a pendulum. This is one of the first intuitive tools I learned to use. To use the body as a pendulum, you ask it yes-or-no questions. You designate your body's forward and backward direction as "yes" or "no," respectively. "Yes" could be when the body leans forward, and "No" when it leans backward.

You can practice this technique with food. Pick a food that is likely healthy for you, such as a green veggie. Hold it at your solar plexus. Do your best not to look for an answer but rather allow the answer to come to you. Does your body lean toward the vegetable? That is a "yes" signal for you. If your body doesn't lean either way, the food might have a neutral effect, or you might need to relax your body more. Next, pick up something unhealthy for you, such as a bag of sugar. Hold it at your solar plexus. Does your body lean toward it or away from it? As you get used to working with your body this way, you can advance to questions about life—but practice the small things first to get the hang of it.

Tune into your body's subtle energy field. I often call the body's subtle energy field the body's "rainbow." To read your energy field, it helps to have a reference point to help set your compass. First, imagine a joyful moment in your life. How does it affect your energy field? Does it brighten it, make it feel lighter and more expansive, open your heart, or maybe all of these? Next, imagine a somewhat sad or frustrating moment. It doesn't have to be the saddest moment in your life. Notice what happens with your field. Does it become dull, heavier, or smaller, possibly shielding your heart? (After calibrating your compass, let yourself reset your emotional state by embracing these emotions as you would hug a baby, just as described in the Four-Step Process for Difficult Emotions on page 47.)

Once you have experienced that comparison—what it feels like to brighten or dull your field—imagine feeling another emotion and compare it with what you have experienced. For example, you could imagine sitting on the couch watching television versus walking in nature. How does your body's energy field feel with each? Different or the same? If different, can you tell what the differences are?

Use your body's senses, symptoms, and physiology to guide your decision-making. What do you feel in your body as you imagine stepping in different directions? Does it tense up, get queasy, or breathe shallow breaths? Or does it relax, breathe easy, and make you smile? You can also combine these observations with what you notice in your subtle energy field (a dulling and contraction, versus a brightening and expansion). Practice this technique with a minor question, such as choosing what to eat at a restaurant. As you look at or touch each menu item, is there one that relaxes your body? Unhealthy cravings will tense up the body despite what your thoughts might say. Be honest with yourself.

Place one or both of your hands on your heart and notice how it feels when you ask specific questions. Whatever rings true or whatever needs tending will create a feeling of heart-opening or expansion. It's your heart saying, "Yes! That's it!" Another way to do this is to place one hand on your forehead and the other on your heart. The touch of your hands helps to connect the electromagnetic fields of both heart and head, like a telephone line. Again, imagine choosing one direction and then another. How does your heart feel? Does your head agree? You might experiment with this technique after you've had a challenging interaction with someone and are unsure how to respond. Strengthening the connection between your heart and mind with your hands will help you see the situation more lovingly. Then, you can respond from love rather than fear.

Fear will be less intimidating once you can use your body as a compass because you'll know how to interpret it. When we no longer fear the fear, it dissipates, and we are grounded and present no matter how we feel. But if we continue to fear the fear, it becomes a self-perpetuating cycle. It's the same with worry, anger, and sadness. When we're no longer worried about being worried, angry about being angry, or sad about being sad, we ground into the body. Understanding our body's language means we always have a compass with us.

Our Triune Nature and Our Health

As your understanding of yourself grows, you may delve deeper into the energetic, intuitive, and spiritual. Regardless of where you are on your journey, it's important to realize we are human beings with a body, a mind, and a spirit. That's the definition of our triune nature: we are three in one. There is a miraculous spark of life in each of these layers. Healing can occur on any of these dimensions, for in truth, all healing is one and comes from the divine. Sometimes, healing is needed for one layer more than another—still, they are all equal. One layer is not better than another in the human experience. Let yourself be human.

Summary:

In this chapter, we discussed your body's innate wisdom and using it for guidance. Learning to use the body's compass takes courage and a desire to know yourself fully.

- Know your constitution. Understanding where you are on the sensitivity gradient helps you use your body like a compass.

- A sensitive person can pick up on the vibes around them. When what you feel does not match what you see, something outside you is out of balance. Consider what you sense as neutral data points so you don't absorb the energy around you.

- There are many types of intuition. Determine which types are more natural for you: intuitive feeling, intuitive seeing, intuitive hearing, intuitive smelling, intuitive knowing, or pure channeling. You can cultivate and strengthen any of these.

- Your body's energy field, or rainbow, reflects your current approach to life.

- When you are no longer afraid of being afraid, the fear dissipates.

- When you learn to use your body as a compass, you can ask it for guidance in your life.

- All healing comes from one divine source and includes healing on multiple dimensions, whether body, mind, or spirit. Let your intuition guide you toward the path of ease.

Sometimes, we can find the path of ease through the body. However, we need to address and integrate body, mind, and spirit at some point. Much of the time, it's the mind that is working against the body, and the body cannot keep up. The mind loves to analyze and can get stuck on the many details. Sensitive people are very good at picking up on the many details. Still, there's the risk of getting distracted by all the subtleties. In other words, let's not lose the forest for the trees. For true balance, our thoughts need to align with the body. In Part 2, we turn our attention to our thoughts and the intuitive mind.

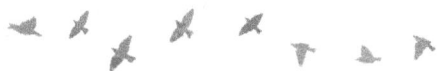

Exercises for the Intuitive Body

Cross-Lateral Movements
(See page 22 in chapter 1 for others.)

Butterfly Hugs
EMDR therapists Lucina Artigas and Ignacio Jarero created this technique for survivors of Hurricane Pauline, which devastated Mexico City in 1998. It's another cross-lateral exercise that helps reconnect the left and right sides of the body through bilateral stimulation.

Here's what's involved. Either cross your hands over your chest or give yourself a big hug. Then, alternate each hand tapping on your chest or your arm depending on how your hands are positioned. Tap slowly and gently as if you were soothing a baby. This kind of slow, alternate tapping acts to cradle your nervous system.

You can then add feel-good mantras such as these:

All is well.

I have courage.

I can let myself be.

Alternating Hand Clasps
You know how people sometimes wring their hands when they're worried? You could think of hand-wringing as the body's attempt to rebalance itself by activating the meridian points in the fingers. In that state, though, the mind can be resistant. So let's make the clasp more productive by aligning mind, body, and spirit.

Alternating Hand Clasps is a mindful exercise combining breath with motion. Start with your hands in prayer position and inhale. Then exhale slowly while clasping your hands. Repeat by inhaling and returning your hands to the prayer position. On the next exhalation, clasp your hands by shifting your fingers the other way.

Figure 3 - Alternating Hand Clasps

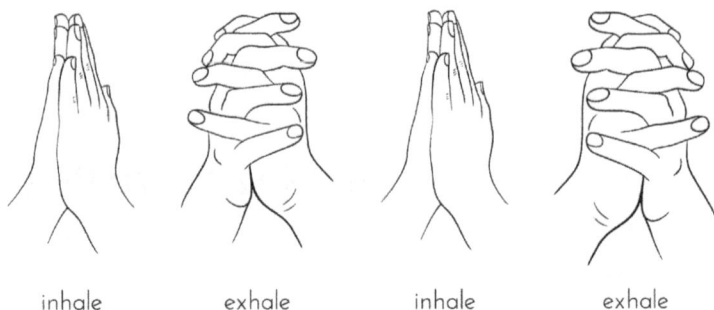

inhale   exhale   inhale   exhale

Humming for Vagal Toning

Humming is a form of vocal toning or sound healing with your voice. Research has shown that humming helps to calm, reduce stress, balance blood pressure, lower heart rate, increase lymph circulation, increase feel-good endorphins, open up the airways, and improve sleep.[1] When we hum, we massage the body with self-created sound waves; the massage also improves the activity of the vagus nerve, which plays a major role in the calming, parasympathetic response. When we hum, a 15 to 20 percent increase of nitrous oxide is released in the airways. Nitrous oxide helps to open up the airways for better breathing.

Take a moment to practice the basics of humming. Keep in mind that humming requires that your nasal passages be open.

1. Stand or sit in a comfortable, neutral position.

2. Take a few deep breaths.

3. Keep your mouth closed and your jaw relaxed.

4. Make an "mmmmmm…" sound.

5. Feel the vibration in your lips, throat, cheeks, and sinus cavities.

6. You might feel vibrations elsewhere in your body. You can also direct the healing vibrations to specific areas, including your subtle energy body. Noticing what you feel will help you develop self-awareness.

7. Continue humming for at least five minutes.

Humming is an easy practice to incorporate into your everyday life. Consider spending at least five minutes humming daily for two weeks to see what you notice. You can hum while sitting in meditation, walking the dog, folding the laundry, picking up the kids, or anytime you think of it.

Writing a Letter to Your Body

Give yourself at least twenty minutes to write a love letter to your body. Every part of your body is precious, so include all the details, from the texture of your skin and your hair, to your muscles, bones, heart, and belly, all your sensory and internal organs, and any hurts or scars—every detail has a story to tell.

When my kids were little, they pounced on my belly and said they loved how squishy it was. I would chuckle to myself because I knew this was a loving compliment, and I would agree with them that my belly was wonderful because it could stretch and carry my beautiful babies.

You can use these writing prompts to give your whole body thanks and love:

Dear Body,

Thank you for . . .

I'm sorry that . . .

I wish that . . .

I accept that . . .

I believe that together, we can . . .

I'd like to tell you that . . .

You are a miracle to me because . . .

Remember that time that . . .

I was scared when you . . .

Sometimes I'm frustrated because . . .

I'm so glad that . . .

I smile when you . . .

I laugh when you . . .

I love that . . .

I promise to . . .

I hope that . . .

I believe in you because . . .

I'm so happy that . . .

I love you because you are my body.

Love,

Me

A Conversation with Your Masculine and Feminine Energies[2]

This exercise helps you understand different aspects of yourself. Imagine an energetic male version and an energetic female version of yourself. These aspects are not gender-based but energetic, and together they represent the whole of yin and yang. This is an opportunity to discover what the energetic masculine and feminine versions of yourself have to say to each other. Give each a turn and hear each one out. Are they willing to speak to each other? Are they on the same page? Does one tend to dominate the conversation? Honor and respect each aspect—each one is part of you. The imaginary conversation can continue until there is a sense of peace between the two and they can hug and thank each other.

It's amazing what can come up when you do this exercise. Often, I find it sounds like a conversation between my husband and me, which is uncanny. This exercise is an enlightening way for me to balance my interior world so that there's more ease in my external world.

A Five-Senses Meditation for Grounding

Bringing awareness to the physical senses helps us stay present in the body. This meditation will include touch, sight, hearing, smell, and taste. If you would like to practice the meditation as you read it, take a moment to pause after each paragraph. You can also record yourself reading it. The cells of your body love to hear your voice. Allowing yourself to be seen and heard by you is powerful healing.

First, notice what gravity feels like. If you're standing, feel how your feet are pulled toward the earth. What does that interface feel like? If you're sitting, feel your legs and buttocks against the chair or surface you're sitting on. Notice a pressure or force where they meet. Gravity is at work here, constantly grounding you. Now, look around you. What do you see? How bright is it? What colors do you see? What shapes? Let your eyes wander and drink in your surroundings. Can you reach out to touch something? What does its texture feel like?

Next, what do you hear? If you're outside, do you hear the wind or other nature sounds? If you're inside, what sounds are in the room? Even when it's quiet, there are sounds in a building or home. Take a moment to notice and breathe in the sounds around you.

Now, notice whether there are any smells, however strong or faint. Take a big inhalation and exhalation to wake up your senses. Awareness of your sense of smell will enhance your intuition.

Finally, bring your curiosity to your taste buds. Whether we're eating or drinking, our tastebuds are still at work. What does your mouth taste like right now? What does the air taste like?

Sometimes, noticing our five senses all at once can create sensory overload. If this is the case for you, take in each of the senses one at a time. With practice, you can become aware of multiple senses and remain in a space of neutral curiosity. You can also combine this meditation with the last exercise in Part 1, Your Rainbow Body on page 84. The ability to experience life through our physical senses is an amazing gift.

Progressive Muscle Relaxation for Body Awareness

Progressive muscle relaxation (PMR) helps develop your awareness of the body as you purposely tense up different body parts, squeezing tightly and then relaxing suddenly. Here's how:

- Shut your eyes tight for a few seconds; then relax them.
- Wrinkle your forehead and face; then relax.
- Shrug your shoulders up high and tight into your neck; then relax.
- Ball up your hands and squeeze them; then relax.
- Squeeze your buttocks; then let go.

- Tense your legs; then relax.

- Curl your toes in tightly for a few seconds; then relax.

- Curl your whole body into a tight ball, hold for a moment, and then relax.

The conscious tensing of different body parts teaches you to bring your attention to the body. Letting go and relaxing afterward lets you experience the difference between feeling tense and relaxed. PMR is a great exercise for learning to be present in your body, recognizing tension early on, and knowing how to relax and let go.

Dancing Organically

I have patients dance when they haven't yet learned the Tension and Trauma Releasing Exercises. Dancing organically gives your body permission to unwind and shake off stress. All you have to do is pick a comfortable location, whether in the privacy of your home or outside in nature, play some music you love, and let your body be moved from within. You are dancing for yourself—this is your own private dance party. Your dance doesn't have to look like a particular kind of dance or choreography. Let your body speak, breathe, and express how it desires through movement. This is an intuitive dance.

Dance creates flow in the body, moving the physical, mental, and emotional dimensions. Consider starting with five minutes each day or every other day in the beginning. If you do that, you could find that amazing things are possible. Emotions may bubble up in various forms, whether laughter or tears. You decide what you're okay with. Depending on the circumstances, one person might be fine with crying, while another is overwhelmed by tears. If you feel overwhelmed or uncomfortable, slow down and take a break. Again, you get to decide what is right for you.

Dancing is a great opportunity for your body to express itself to you, and when you bring awareness to the movement, you align the mind, body, and spirit. Pent-up emotions and tension can start to unwind. Feeling stuck or frustrated? Dancing is a simple and effective way to get back in the flow.

Opening and Centering the Heart Field

This is one of my favorite exercises for opening and centering the heart field on multiple dimensions. The first part of the exercise energetically opens the vertical (or longitudinal) midline to release tension and shock in the body. Opening up the midline is an important part of the osteopathic treatment, and I'll do this for most every patient that comes to see me. In this exercise, you'll open up the energetic flow of your midline using your breath and awareness.

Step 1. First, imagine the sun and heavens shining love on you in a brilliant white light. This white light shines down through the crown of your head and down through your head, neck, and shoulders. Pause at the heart center as it's filled with this light and love from the heavens. Stay here for at least a few slow and easy breaths. Breathe in the light.

Then, continue letting the light and love flow down your arms, downward through your solar plexus, down through your abdomen, your hips and pelvis, down your legs, knees, and ankles, and through the bottoms of your feet, deep into the earth. Pause there for a moment, and let the heavens give love and thanks to the earth through you. Breathe it in slowly.

Then, let that light and love from the earth come back up through the soles of your feet as if your feet were roots drinking up nourishment from the earth. Let that light and love continue upward through your ankles and knees, your thighs, hips, and pelvis, your abdomen and solar plexus, and your heart. Pause here again, and let your heart be filled with light for as long as you need. Breathe it in. Then, raise your arms up, and let the light and love flow up your arms to your hands, up from your heart, through your neck and throat, up through your third eye and your crown, to the heavens. Let the earth send love and thanks to the heavens through you. Breathe this in slowly.

Step 2. Now, imagine your heart field opening out in front of you and behind you. If the front of your heart represented the future and the back of it the past, let yourself balance in the center of the heart field where the present moment is. You could imagine a string running through the heart field being tugged at the front and the back, by the future and past. See if you can balance that tension equally on both sides, so your heart is situated in the neutral center. The neutral center is where you can access the "omnipotential" of your being. Pause and breathe here with easy, slow breaths.

Step 3. Next, imagine your heart field expanding to the right and left sides. Remember, the right side tends to represent masculine energy while the left side tends to represent feminine energy. Let the two sides come into balance. You could imagine another string running through the heart that tugs from the right and left sides. See if you can balance the tension and bring your heart to neutral center. In this state, you are open, aware, and a powerful source of love. Pause again, and breathe this in with easy, slow breaths. Bask in this open heart field, balanced above and below, in front and behind, and on either side. Feel the radiance beam out from your heart center in all directions, like a bright star. Here you'll find the confidence to create what you desire with love from love. After all, we *are* love.

Detangling Your Cords

You have energetic cords connecting you to everything and everyone in your life. They are constantly changing, and some are meant to be temporary. And sometimes, there can be an entanglement, which feels like your energy is tangled up with someone else's. You know there's an entanglement when you're bothered and can't stop thinking about the person, place, or thing. Maybe you've had an argument or are having a hard time getting along. Maybe you're overly concerned about what a certain person might think. The entanglement drains energy from both sides.

Rather than cutting these tangled cords, which is a way of cutting the person, thing, or place out of your life, I like to detangle the cords and create more clarity for both sides. Then, you can choose how you hope to move forward for more peaceful relationships. I like to detangle my cords after any difficult interaction and at the end of each day. When I do this, I feel a wave of peace wash over my mind and body.

The amazing thing is it also helps the other person because we are all connected. Just before writing this, I practiced detangling cords for a patient I was worried about. She was upset about something, and I didn't feel we had enough time to talk it through during her appointment. Minutes after I did this practice, she emailed me to let me know all was well.

Here are four variations for detangling cords. See what feels best for you.

Imagine the many cords reaching out from you to everyone and everything in your life. These energetic cords are typically connected to your midline energy center, though that is not an absolute. Now, imagine gently zipping up all these cords so that your energy returns to you and the energy that belongs to the other side is returned there, to the person, place, or thing. You can simply think or say, "Zip!" and know it is done. I learned this exercise from a friend and colleague, Deborah Craydon, an energy healer and flower essence practitioner.

If it's difficult to imagine zipping these cords, ask the Stillness to do it for you, and trust it is done.

Sometimes, the idea of zipping up cords doesn't sit well with some people, especially the cords to their loved ones. Again, detangling cords is not necessarily about removing people from your life but clarifying the relationship. Another visual you could try is imagining the cord as a hollow tube. Shine white light through the tube so it shines crystal clear; this way, your cord is made of pure light, and any ripples are smoothed out.

Another way to do this detangling is to imagine a sphere of love surrounding the entanglement as shown in Figure 4 below. Imagine yourself hugging the cord bundle as if it were a hurt child. Create a field of loving-kindness around the cord bundle. You might say a sincere "thank you" and "I love you" to soften the tangled energies. If the two ends of the cords were hands, would they be gripping, fisted, or pushing? Imagine the hands loosening to free each other.

Figure 4 - Placing a Sphere Around an Entanglement

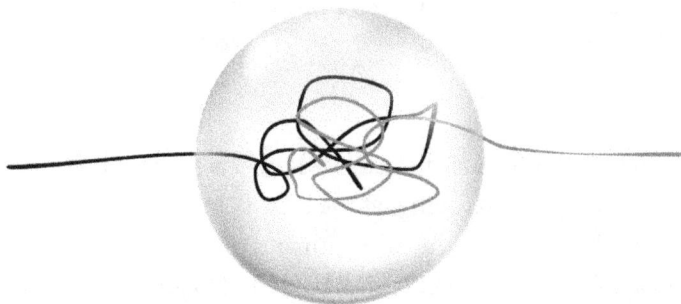

Massaging Your Energy Field

The hands are amazing healing tools. *Your* hands are amazing healing tools. There are many meridian points (an acupuncture term for energy points) on your palms, and you can wake them up. You can do this by briskly rubbing your palms together, the way you would warm up your hands. Bring your awareness to your hands as they warm up; as you do so, you heighten your hands' sensing abilities. The palms can act as another set of eyes or antennas.

Next, gently comb through your energy field with your hands about six to twelve inches past your physical body. Move your hands as if you were smoothing out your energy field all around your body, starting from the top of your field and working down to its bottom. You're giving yourself a subtle energy massage, brushing off the static in your field. You might notice little ripples, spikes, or tangles in some areas more than others. These represent static in your field. No need to be alarmed—simply smooth these out with your palms, gently brushing through your field to smooth out the static. You can also shake your hands toward the earth to ground the excess charge. Imagine shaking them over a compost pile, where the excess charge can transform into something nourishing. Notice how you feel after a few minutes of this subtle energy massage.

Your Rainbow Body and Three Variations on a Body Scan

Have you noticed that when people are joyful and peaceful, their eyes sparkle and they look like they're glowing? That's because their subtle energy body *is* glowing! I like to call the energy body our rainbow. It's also known as your aura. In this whole-body scan, you'll practice tuning into both your physical and energetic bodies to be more fully present. Your body needs your love and attention. Go ahead and give it what it needs.

Body Scan 1

First, get into a comfortable position, whether sitting, standing, or lying down. Then, as if you're gazing at the sunset, bring a gentle awareness to your breathing. Notice the in-breath and the out-breath. Just notice. How does it feel? Just say hello to the breath. No judgment.

Now, bring your awareness to your entire physical body. At first, you may not be able to take it all in, and that's okay. See how your body is as you start to bring awareness to it. Your body has been waiting for your love and attention.

And now imagine that your physical body is made of light and stardust. See what that feels like. Are any areas lighter than others? Could some be filled with more light? If so, imagine you're sprinkling stardust on the areas that could use more light. What you find is not about judging it as good or bad. This is about tending to your body, giving it what it needs—giving love to your body.

Next, expand your awareness to include your subtle energy body, your rainbow body. Imagine your rainbow body glowing with its light all around you. Just notice this. Notice without any concern about good or bad. Is your subtle energy body symmetric? Are there areas that could use more light? If so, sprinkle them with stardust. Sprinkle stardust all through your rainbow body, and really let it sparkle. It's just like taking care of your home. Sometimes the subtle energy body can get cluttered and congested, just like the physical body. But with gentle, loving awareness, you can take care of it.

If some areas feel like they need to be swept, imagine sweeping them with a little energy broom or a light wand. You can transform anything in your field into something more beneficial by consciously filling it with light and love and letting your rainbow body shine.

Do a scan from head to toe. It doesn't have to take long, but you don't have to rush either. As you scan, are there areas that could use some love today? Where is calling to you? Go there. Give it a big hug. Use your light wand and stardust to transform it with light. That's what we're made of; we are made of the same elements as stardust.

Body Scan 2
Do the same body scan exercise, but instead of feeling into your body, imagine that your body is in front of you. This approach works well for people who are visual and don't feel in touch with their bodies.

Body Scan 3
Another way to do this body scan is by coloring your body. You draw

a loose outline of your body—it might look like a gingerbread person—and then color in the different body parts, from head to toe, in whatever way you feel would best represent how you feel. You could also color in your energy body that extends beyond your physical body. Again, there's no right or wrong to this exercise. Don't overthink it. Afterward, you'll have a map of your intuitive body.

Figure 5 - Gingerbread Body and Aura for Coloring

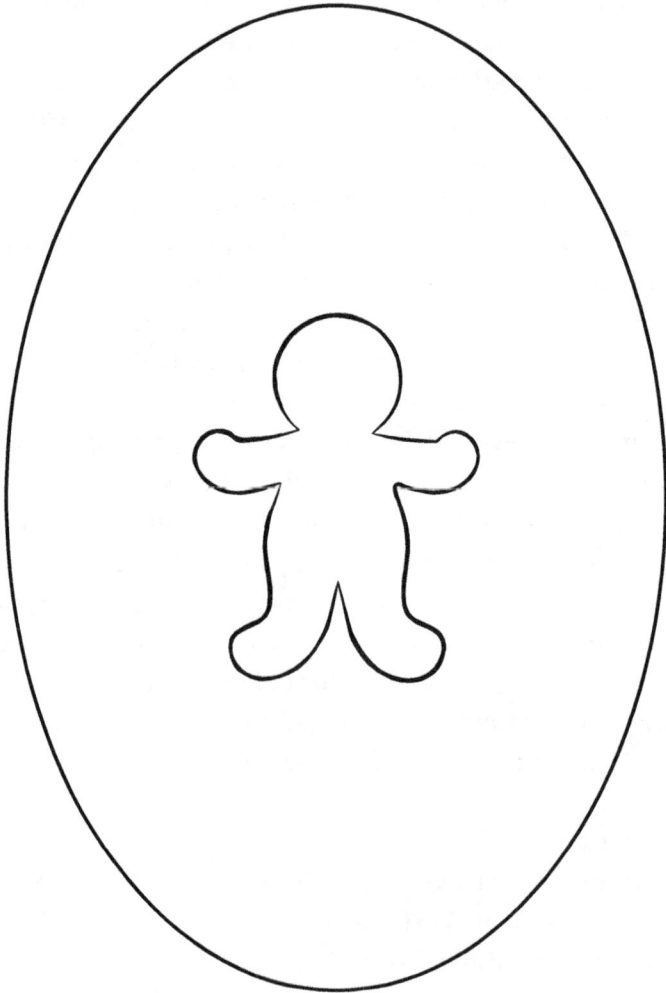

PART II

The Intuitive Mind

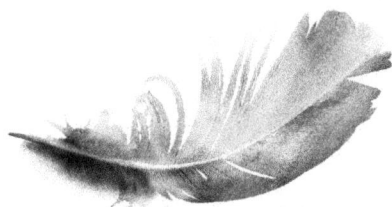

This was the hardest part of the book to write, which is easy to understand because the mind is the part of our being that tends to get in the way of the intuitive body and the intuitive spirit. The mind second-guesses, hesitates, and doubts our true nature. Like spirit, our minds are infinite, but we often need to be reminded of this. You might have heard the advice "get out of your own way" when your mind was sabotaging or blocking you from accessing your dreams.

Various exercises are scattered throughout the next three chapters, with additional exercises at the end of the section. Do the ones that seem simple and easy first. This will help you get out of the mindset that you have to work very hard to take the steps of healing. Yes, it does take energy to shift gears and change, but why take on the hard stuff when you haven't tended to what's easy first?

Get ready to dive into the intuitive mind!

CHAPTER 4

THOUGHTS—WHAT ARE THEY?

"Your thoughts are the energy that help shape your reality."

In my first year of medical school, I had an incredible idea: Instead of comparing everything to the placebo effect, why don't we study it? Why don't we harness the body's innate capacity to get better?

A placebo is a pretend treatment, such as a sugar pill used as "a control" in standardized studies for comparison with the "real" treatment. It's how the gold standard of studies—the double-blind placebo-controlled trial—is set up. Neither the patients nor the physicians giving the treatment know whether a patient is getting the actual treatment (usually a drug) or the placebo. Hence, the term "double-blind." However, according to a Harvard study led by Ted Kaptchuk, researchers found that even when a placebo pill was labeled and patients knew what they were being given, the placebo was 50 percent as effective as the drug in reducing migraine pain.[1]

I couldn't wait to share my radical yet common-sense idea with my friends and colleagues. I believed this could change everything! I'm not sure what I expected, but at the very least, I thought they would be curious and that we'd have a lively discussion. I had no idea how far outside the box the idea was at the time. My attending physician cocked his head to the side when I told him and said, "Well, that's an interesting way to look at it." And that was the end of the conversation. I looked around at the other medical students, but they weren't looking at me—they were looking at the attending physician. Without further ado, we moved on to whatever the next topic was. If the physicians and physicians-in-training weren't interested in the body's mysterious ability to heal on its own, then who was? My heart fell.

I was sure I wasn't the only one with this idea. At the time, though, I decided to lay low since there was already so much to study and keep up with. I was perplexed by the lack of interest, just as I was when I told my medical ethics class about Doris. There's so much more we are capable of if only we open our minds to it.

Four years later, during my pediatric residency in the Bronx, I happened upon Dr. Andrew Weil's book *Spontaneous Healing*. In chapter 3, he talks about the placebo effect. I was over the moon! I had found a community of like-minded physicians and researchers interested in the workings of the placebo effect's healing powers. The following table summarizes several factors thought to contribute to the placebo effect.

Table 9 - Factors Influencing the Placebo Effect

Factors Influencing the Placebo Effect	Details
Subconscious Conditioned Response	A bit like Pavlov's dog: You ring a bell each time you give the dog food. After a while, the dog starts salivating when it hears the bell. Maybe you associate taking a pill with pain relief, so taking a fake medication could still cause you to feel better.
Conscious Expectation	If you believe a specific treatment will help you, it's more likely that it will. The mind is a powerful thing. When we're aware of the mind's capabilities, we can use it to help shape our reality.
Social Factors	A support system of people who care about and believe in you also encourages your belief in yourself. In addition, a group of people whose thoughts and purpose are aligned can also have a healing effect, encouraging your mind to believe in yourself.

Understanding certain terms related to your thoughts and consciousness will help you better understand the placebo effect and how to use it to your benefit.

Mind, Consciousness, and Intention

Have you ever thought about how the mind, consciousness, and intention are different from one another? It's come up in various classes I've taken, from philosophy to neuroscience to cranial osteopathy. Even if you're not so into the esoteric, bear with me because these questions are about our very existence.

What is the mind? There are so many meanings, but I'd like us to look at the definition from cognitive psychology. In my work as a physician, I use this definition because it is important for me to be able to communicate with mental health professionals, as well as other healthcare professionals. Although I do recognize other valuable interpretations of the mind from other philosophies and studies, for the purposes of clarity in this book, let's continue with what's been both helpful and accessible in my medical practice. Cognitive psychologists define the mind as "an information processor" and study how we take information from the outside world and make sense of it.[2] The information processing that goes on in the mind includes perception, attention, language, memory, thinking, and awareness.

Where is the mind? There is no exact answer to this question. Scientists and, long before them, philosophers have pondered this question for millennia. Quite simply, we don't know the answer. Typically, the brain is considered the organ of the mind, although the brain and the mind are different.[3] Some scientists use a computer-based analogy to explain how the mind works. Neurologist Ennapadam Krishnamoorthy writes, "The mind . . . is a virtual entity, one that reflects the workings of the neural networks, chemical and hormonal systems in our brain."[4] In other words, like a computer storing and processing information, the mind is not in any one place but an association of networks.

This understanding of the mind is complicated even more by the mystery of consciousness and the soul. In psychology, the definition of consciousness is often limited to the cognitive domain and does not consider the soul. In this book, however, I will use an expanded definition of consciousness that includes an awareness of the soul. As one neuroscientist told me, these are topics that scientists avoid like the plague yet wonder about at night. Mind, consciousness, and soul are too much, too big, too infinite to be defined by science as we know it. Perhaps, as neuroscientist Dr. Karen Rommelfanger has suggested, science is not the domain we use to study and understand consciousness.[5]

I'm okay with that for now, and I'm okay with the fact that science—at least our current scientific understanding—does not have the answers to everything. I deeply respect and trust the inner workings of the universe. It seems impossible for us to know it all. The universe is infinite, while our human experience seems finite. Still, the more we understand our consciousness and mind, the more we can co-create our lives with our consciousness, mind, and body attuned with the oneness of the universal Spirit.

As I see it, our minds are an incredible tool for living. Our minds can generate thoughts that can help us create our human experience. When conscious of our thoughts, we can consciously steer the direction of our lives. When unaware of our thoughts, we function like a machine on autopilot. In autopilot mode, subconscious stress and trauma patterns run our lives. You might notice this when you have negative thought loops. When you think and act without consciousness, the mind can run away with itself instead of being anchored in the heart center. It will run old programming that doesn't update to the current situation. There will be incongruencies as the body and spirit will constantly be sending messages that something is off balance and needs recalibrating. We hope to be more aware of ourselves so that we can choose what we think. That's where the fun is!

Next, what is intention? Intention is purposeful thought. Intention on its own, however, is not alive. Think of a robot with a specific purpose. It can follow instructions and decode new information, but a robot cannot be alive. Consciousness is needed to be alive—and to truly live—which brings me to a more succinct description of consciousness. As I noted earlier, consciousness is the awareness of your soul. We will discuss the soul more in Part 3, but for now, know that your soul is all love. This means that consciousness—awareness of the soul—is a loving awareness. In short, *consciousness is love.*

In this human experience, your soul (love) desires to express itself in physical reality. How does your soul get that love out into the world? Through intention (purposeful thought), which acts as a vector for expressing love. A loving intention is both feeling-thinking love. This is how we create in the world: Love + Intention = Creation. Why does intention need love to create? Love remembers that we are all part of the oneness. Love centers the creative process and automatically guides the mind to consider the good of all because love realizes the ripple effects of our actions. Love is the realization of oneness. Love is consciousness.

The creative process is life in balance. To better understand, let's explore love and intention without each other. Love without intention is passive. Love (the conscious awareness of the soul) desires to be expressed. Without intention, love is still omnipotent but not put into action. To feel fully alive as a human, we must put love into action. We must live love, and loving intention makes that possible. Also, intention without love is not creative but destructive, tearing things down instead of building them up. Sometimes, creation does require transmutation or a literal change in form to create anew, but that's different from destruction. I think of how mushrooms help decompose organic matter and return it to the soil to nourish new growth. That's not destruction but change that renews.

Here's a table to keep you on track as we continue. (Don't get too bogged down in the terms. Let their meanings digest into something meaningful for you, even if your descriptions differ from mine.)

Definitions of Terms

As with my definition of the mind, I realize many schools of thought provide definitions of the terms listed here based on their understanding. See Table 10 on the next page for the definitions we'll be working with in this book.

Note that I've added the term *subconscious* to the table. Your subconscious is below your conscious awareness. It can function with unprocessed trauma patterns; however, your subconscious also has

Table 10 - Working Definitions of Mind, Thought, and Consciousness[6]

Term	Description
Mind	Generates thoughts
Ego-Mind	Learned patterns of thoughts, ideas, and beliefs (See chapter 5)
Thought	Tool to create the human experience
Intention	Purposeful thought
Light	Divine guidance, intuition (See chapters 7 and 10)
Subconscious	Below conscious awareness
Consciousness	Awareness of the soul, Love
Conscious Intention	Loving thought with the highest purpose
Love	Consciousness, the realization of Oneness
Creation	Love + Intention

access to your intuition. How? Your subconscious can take information in from multiple physical and nonphysical dimensions, which is more information than you can consciously think about at one time. Still, there are ways to bring your subconscious impulses to your conscious awareness. The exercises in Parts 2 and 3 of this book can help.

To review, when you think and act without consciousness (love), the mind can run away with itself and away from the heart center. A mind without heart is like a machine running on autopilot, running old programming, including trauma programming, that doesn't update to the current situation. It's impossible to feel whole this way because the body and spirit will be out of balance with the mind; they will communicate this imbalance through symptoms of physical discomfort, fear, or anxiety. Remember that nature loves balance. So, though the imbalance might be destructive, it's also telling you where the healing is—in grounding and returning to the heart center, attuning your body, mind, and spirit.

To regain balance, it helps to have self-awareness. When specific thought patterns have been dominant, it takes energy to shift out of them. A gentle, loving awareness of your thoughts can give you that momentum at any moment. (No wonder the energy needed to move or shift is called "momentum"—it's a moment-to-moment phenomenon.) If you need help grounding and centering, get help from a qualified professional. Taking the time to tend to your inner world is worthwhile and vital. The world becomes your playground once you start living consciously and choose purposeful, heart-centered thoughts (intentions).

How Thoughts Become Things

Your thoughts are the energy that helps shape your reality. In the words of Edgar Cayce: "Spirit is the Life, Mind is the Builder, the Physical is the Result." Edgar Cayce was the most studied 20th-century psychic and is often called "the father of holistic medicine." He emphasized that the mind's role is creative and that ideas first spark in spirit—hence, the term *inspiration*. However, for our ideas to take physical form, we need our thoughts. Our thoughts are the energetic vibration that leads to action and physical results.

Again, your loving awareness (consciousness) is key. We see the importance of awareness in the double-slit experiment. The scientist Thomas Young first set up the double-slit experiment in 1804 to study whether light behaves as a particle or a wave. He sent a beam of light through two slits in a plate to see where the light beams landed on a screen behind the plate. If light had a particle nature (photons), it would create two straight lines on the screen corresponding to the two slits—but if light had a wave-like nature, then an interference pattern would show graduated dark and light bands on the screen.

Which pattern did the experiment show, a particle or a wave? The results were wacky. When the scientists observed the experiment directly (or set up a measurement device to observe the light passing through the slit), the light created two discrete lines on the screen—corresponding to a particle nature. However, when the experiment was left to run on its own, the light made a wave pattern on the screen. Basically, any conscious observation of the experiment changed the light's behavior from wave-like to particle-like. Although there's been much debate about the how and why of this phenomenon, the mystery remains. This uncertainty, this mystery, is also one of life's delights. Somehow, our consciousness matters, and it helps to shape reality.

One of the first times the significance of this concept struck me was at a Matrix Energetics workshop taught by Richard Bartlett and Melissa Joy. Richard Bartlett is a chiropractor and naturopath renowned for his work in quantum healing. Melissa Joy is Dr. Bartlett's longtime co-teacher. She has a master's degree in neuroscience and psychology and a knack for explaining the complexities of quantum physics in digestible bites. Here are a few key steps based on the healing concepts Richard and Melissa teach.[7]

1. Ground and center yourself in your heart to tap into your loving awareness (consciousness). You can use the exercise on page 81: Opening and Centering the Heart Field.

2. Create a loving intention by choosing where to place your loving awareness. There's a popular saying, "Where you focus grows." So, if you focus on illness, all you will see is illness. If you focus on health, you will expand your perception of health. It's not ignoring one or the other but *choosing* where you'd like to direct your energy.

3. Let go of the outcome. A shift is more likely to occur when you focus on health with conscious, loving intentions and then let go of the outcome. Similar to the scientists *not* observing the double-slit experiment, when you look away, the particle becomes a wave.

When Richard Bartlett taught us how to do this for ourselves, reality seemed to bend. His techniques blended with what I had learned as a cranial osteopath. They became a part of me and sped up my treatments.

Once, a young ice hockey player named Barry came to see me with an injured hip. He had already been to an orthopedist who recommended rest. Although nothing serious was found, Barry was left limping for weeks. When I saw him, he had many minor strains in the muscle and fascia, which wasn't surprising for a hockey player. About thirty minutes into the treatment, I didn't feel I was making much progress, and Barry still felt pain in his hip. Then I remembered Richard Bartlett's statement: "Let go of the outcome." So I told myself, *I'd like Barry to feel better, but I don't know what will happen. I accept all outcomes. It is up to something greater than me.* It was my truth, and I fully accepted it. Lo and behold, after another ten minutes or so, Barry's hip released, and he felt like himself again. No pain and no limp.

I tell you this story because you can approach things this way, too. In short:

- Center in your heart.
- Make a conscious, loving intention.
- Let go of the outcome.

By setting a conscious intention, you are directing reality. By letting go, you are allowing your reality to shift and take on a new shape. In other words, you are leaving room for miracles.

Miracles

I love the topic of miracles. What we call "miracles" are simply things we don't yet understand. I see them every day in my office: *each person is a miracle.* The world is made of miracles—often taken for granted.

Once, I saw a gastroenterologist write the word "miracle" on his final consultation note. A girl named Bella I had been seeing had a history of chronic constipation since birth. Sometimes, she had a bowel movement just once in a month. She would be doubled over in pain, unable to talk comfortably, and had no appetite. If you've ever been constipated, you know how difficult this is. Bella's mom did not give up. She sought integrative and holistic care in addition to regular appointments with the gastroenterologist. Combining remedies that included dietary changes, herbals, and osteopathic treatment to balance the nerve communication and blood flow to her colon helped Bella to start getting better. Over the months, she improved steadily.

Then, one day, Bella and her mom brought me a note from the gastroenterologist: "Miracle! Discharged from GI clinic." The gastroenterologist could not explain what happened—Bella's constipation had been resolved. Fortunately, Bella's mom had left room for a miracle. It was that initial hope that played a part.

From an integrative and holistic health perspective, we better understand what helped Bella. Was it a miracle? Yes and no, depending on how you look at it. Yes, in that no one can predict exactly what will happen. After all, everyone is unique, and you can never be certain how someone might respond to a treatment. On the other hand, we did have a more holistic understanding of gut health and applied what we knew.

If something appears to be a miracle, I recommend taking steps to understand it. I hope that more physicians will take such steps as well. There may be ways to recreate those miracles. What have we got to lose?

Opening to Beginner's Mind

When you look at everything as a miracle, you're always starting from a beginner's mind. It's that fresh perspective as if you were newly born into the universe. You don't know what to expect, and you have no expectations. You aren't burdened by the "what was" or the "cannots."

With a beginner's mind, there's a marvel and appreciation for all that is and an opening to infinite potential. Zen monk Shunryu Suzuki wrote, "In the beginner's mind, there are many possibilities; in the expert's mind, there are few."[8] At the end of the day, there are so many unknowns that no human can claim to know it all. The framework of what we already know is the lens for how we see things, and it typically interferes with how we take in new information. Naturally, as we learn new things, we want to fit them into the box of what we know—but what if you learn something new that doesn't fit into your "known" box? You might call that "mind-blown."

Think of a new baby. Before the "stranger anxiety" stage, a baby will smile at you even if the baby doesn't know you. When my youngest daughter was a baby, her sister said, "Mommy, she loves everybody! Even strangers! Even if you're good or bad!" Babies have no judgment, only love, an unconditional agape love. Babies also love their bodies, sounds, and interactions with the world. Everything is new and interesting. It's a marvelous way to explore and learn.

When you look at the world this way, you create an opening for new ways of thinking. You don't limit yourself to what you already know. Albert Einstein said, "You can't solve a problem with the same thinking you used to create it." To innovate, we must be open to possibilities, including what we don't yet know. With a constant return to the beginner's mind, you can allow that flow of openness to continue. I like to tap into a beginner's mind consciously anytime I hope to learn something new. I realize everyone has a unique perspective, so even when I may not initially agree with someone's point of view, I listen and attempt to understand their perspective.

As you practice opening your mind, you will have more thoughts to choose from. Imagine the ocean's constant waves. Like those waves, thoughts emerge naturally from an ocean of infinite potential. Which thought waves would you like to surf? Choose wisely because water can carry messages through time and space.

Messages in Water

We are made up of mostly water—about 60 percent by weight and volume for adults—and when we look at the number of water molecules per all the molecules in the body, the percentage goes way up. About 99 percent of the body's molecules are water molecules because water molecules are smaller than other molecules in the body.[9] These numbers tell you something about the significance of water in our lives.

One of the most magnificent properties of water is that it can hold messages. The late Masaru Emoto conducted experiments to understand the nature of water better.[10] He asked different people to infuse different messages into various containers of water using their thoughts. They did this through intentional thought or meditation. Emoto then put the water samples on little dishes and froze them. When he looked at the frozen samples under a microscope, he observed their crystal formations as they warmed up under the microscope's light. Each was unique, like snowflakes.

Different water crystals formed depending on the thoughts transmitted to the water samples. For example, when "I love you" was the message conveyed to various water samples, similar water crystals took shape among them, even when the message was transmitted in different languages. This also occurred with other messages, such as "Thank you" or "You can do it!" You could see the intention of the words represented in the appearance of the crystals. Loving messages resulted in beautiful water crystal formations, while messages of anger produced disorganized and chaotic formations.[9]

Emoto went on to collaborate with other researchers. He reached out to Lynne McTaggart, an author and researcher who writes and lectures about the power of intention, and invited her to Japan for a water experiment. They asked a large group of people to send loving intentions to a polluted body of water. The before and after photos of the water crystals show that the formation changed from chaotic to organized and beautiful.

These water experiments have so many implications for our lives. Our thoughts are silent intentions that the water in our bodies hear and hold. They are vibrational waves that the water in our bodies amplifies. That's why becoming more conscious of our thoughts and what we hope to create is so important. Water can carry our intentions through time and space. In fact, we are drinking the same water molecules our ancestors drank, which means water can pass on their messages to us. At the same time, we are also sending messages to future generations with the water we leave behind. Consider the messages we send to our children and the future when we pollute the oceans and rivers. We have a choice right now: we can send messages of beauty and love to help restore the earth to its natural beauty for ourselves and all beings.

Here's how you can infuse the water you drink with messages:

1. Pour yourself a glass of water. Consider taking a sip as a baseline to see what you notice about the water.

2. Ground and center in your heart (see the heart-centering exercise on page 81).

3. Hold the glass of water in your hands while holding a loving intention. You can simply think, say or feel, "I love you."

4. Breathe in your loving intention, hold it for a moment, and with a quick outbreath through the nostrils, direct your loving intention to the water.[11]

5. Slowly sip the water and notice what you feel and taste. Is it the same or different than it was when you first poured the water? There is no right or wrong answer, just a practice of loving awareness.

When I infuse the water I drink with love messages, I find it more hydrating and nourishing. The water also tastes smoother, like higher-quality water. It's okay if you don't notice any changes. Trust that the messages you infused in your water are there.

Is this phenomenon true? Is it a placebo? It's both. Water can hold messages, *and* you can take advantage of the placebo effect. We are all connected through water. Our thoughts can affect water. So, let's choose thoughts that are inspired.

Thoughts Are Prayers

You can think of each thought as a prayer—to the Oneness, God, Source, the Divine, the Universe, or whatever word you use for the source of all creation. The more we think about something, the more likely it is to manifest, especially if an authentic emotion magnetizes the thought. Sincerity turns up the loudspeakers of our thought-prayers and sends them out into the universe. So, what wavelengths are you broadcasting right now?

When our thoughts run away from us, we might ask for things we didn't mean. For example, my friend Maxine once asked for a new home but didn't want to move. Boom! A few months later, a tornado hit her house (while she was in it!) Fortunately, she wasn't physically hurt, though she did have to move into temporary housing. The insurance company rebuilt her home like new! You never know how your prayers will be answered, so be clear with your thought-prayers.

Sometimes, I hear people say they wish they could take a loved one's pain and suffering away by taking it on themselves. Parents do this so easily when their child is sick, thinking, *I wish it were me instead.* However, we don't have to wish pain and suffering on ourselves to help someone else feel better. If you notice yourself thinking this way, it's okay. Simply retract and transmute such thoughts. Just because you thought something in the past doesn't mean you can't change it now. All you have to do is retract your thoughts, change them, and be sincere about it.

One way to do this is with the Resetting Your Compass exercise (in Part 1). Send the following words to the Oneness, the Divine, God, whichever term you use:

I'm sorry about the thoughts I sent before.

They were not aligned with my highest self.

I choose to retract any thoughts that do not serve my highest purpose,

And transmute them into pure expressions of love.

I also forgive myself for these thoughts,

As I realize that they are a part of my soul's journey.

I am a child of the Oneness; no matter what I do, say, or think, the Universe always loves me.

Thank you for always listening and understanding me.

I often do this at the beginning of the day and at the end of the day as well. I check in with my thoughts and feelings. If there's anything I'd like to shift, I thank myself for how I am at that moment, and then I choose to transmute the thoughts that are no longer needed.

Once you realize how powerful your thoughts are, you can use them to reclaim your life. In other words, use your thoughts wisely. It's so easy to get caught in a thought loop. When that happens, you're also likely to get stuck in a behavior loop, such as too much TV, social media, drinking, food, arguing, complaining, etc. Basically, too much of anything. But you can choose to start using your thoughts consciously to take charge of your life and align it with your heart and soul.

Whether you are conscious of them or not, thoughts are prayers. You can decide to become aware of them. We'll continue discussing how to do this in the rest of Part 2.

Summary

Your thoughts are the energy that helps shape our reality. To understand this concept, we expanded our definition of what thoughts are.

1. Part of the placebo effect involves the mind's conscious expectation.

2. Your mind is nonlocal—it doesn't have an exact physical address. Thoughts and intentions (purposeful thoughts) are tools of creation. Consciousness is awareness of the soul.

3. To get out of autopilot mode, we must wake up and become conscious of our thoughts.

4. By setting a conscious intention, you are directing reality. Your awareness combined with your thoughts shifts reality. As Edgar Cayce taught, "Spirit is the life, mind is the builder, and the physical is the result."

5. Miracles are phenomena we don't fully understand—yet.

6. Use a beginner's mind to see the world in a new light.

7. Water can hold and amplify thought-messages through time and space.

8. Thoughts become things because each thought is a prayer.

9. Retract and transmute thoughts that you don't mean.

Now that you are thinking about your thoughts and practicing a beginner's mind to open to opportunities, you might feel resistance, an inner tug-of-war going on. In the next chapter, we will look at how the ego-mind creates this internal battle and how we can stop the tug-of-war.

CHAPTER 5

GROUNDING THE MIND

"To work with your mind, you have to be friends with it."

Your ego-mind is a learned pattern of thoughts, ideas, and beliefs based on your life experiences. It's what was impressed upon you as a child by your family, school, community, circumstances, society, and culture. It can be a setup for stereotypes and prejudices. The ego-mind's purpose is to protect you from the world, and it uses your automatic responses to keep you in the box of the known. The ego-mind has a certain rigidity; it likes the security of certainty. This is how it functions.

You can basically think of the ego-mind as your programming. If you want to switch programs, it's time to wake up to your intuition. It's much easier to shift gears when you're aware of your mental programming. We'll look at how you can do that in this chapter.

Your ego-mind is not bad. I hope to make that clear. People sometimes get so down about their stuck patterns, but remember, these patterns are part of a coping mechanism. The ego-mind is trying to help you, albeit in a limited way. So you can thank it for helping you get to where you are now—after all, you're still here. To tap into our limitless nature, we begin with some understanding and compassion for the ego-mind.

Let's back up and look at who you are from a grander perspective. When you became human, your infinite light-being joined with a finite body. As a human being, you are equipped with an ego-mind to help you make sense of the paradox of being human, of being the infinite and the finite combined. Through your interactions with the world, the ego-mind starts to categorize "the way things are." It compares in order to create a self-image, which helps you feel secure because you think you know who you are. An imbalance occurs, however, when you believe you are your ego-mind. Then, when anything threatens the ego-mind's self-image, you'll do anything to protect it. You feel that if you don't maintain the ego-mind's self-image, you will, in a sense, die. So the ego-mind activates survival instincts to save "you."

At its best, you can count on the ego-mind's drive for self-preservation to keep you from walking into oncoming traffic. The ego-mind is not good or bad. What's important is whether it's grounded and balanced. The ego-mind is ungrounded when it believes the self-image it created is all that you are. Therein lies the imbalance because, in truth, you are not your ego-mind.

Your soul remembers that you are a divine light being. Once you understand your ego-mind, it can be a tool for your well-being. You can attune (or harmonize) your ego-mind with your soul's messages. When you nourish your ego-mind with the soul's inner truths, your self-image will be based on who you really are instead of comparisons with the outside world. When the ego-mind says something to you like, "Don't say that," or "Don't do that because people won't like you," you can pause and listen for your heart and soul to direct you. Your heart and soul might tell the ego-mind that it can speak your truth and be kind at the same time.

In this way, you understand your ego-mind, appreciate its drive to keep you safe, *and* you allow yourself to grow beyond its limits and start to change your narrative.

Aha! Moments

You might well experience moments when the ego-mind has a sudden realization of your true self. These moments of insight are called "aha moments." I love to ask people about the aha moments that supported their healing. This is Melinda's story.

Melinda was brand new to holistic health and cranial osteopathy. Although she knew me from our community, coming to me for treatment wasn't exactly in her comfort zone. I explained to her a bit about the process before beginning the hands-on therapy of cranial osteopathy. Working on Melinda, I discovered her rhythms were tense and resistant to change. It was slow-going at first. Five minutes into the treatment, she declared, "I feel awkward!"

"That's okay," I told her. "Let yourself feel awkward."

This was a normal response to a new situation.

Things shifted as soon as Melinda let go of her resistance to feeling awkward. When she gave up the tug-of-war between the unease in her emotional body and her mind's resistance, the flow of Melinda's energy and physical fluids began to increase. And the moment she let go, she felt the improved flow in her body. "I can feel that!" she said and described a tingling sensation moving down her legs as she became more grounded. When she relaxed and released tension, Melinda was able to access healing.

The key to Melinda's healing was not with me. It was within her. Melinda's body-mind-spirit aligned. Despite the initial awkwardness, Melinda shifted into the flow when let herself be. It was a huge aha moment for her. She realized that the ease in healing is *not* in the trying but in dropping resistance and accepting whatever she is feeling is in the moment.

Start Where You Are

It's common for people to spend much of their time wanting to be different, trying to be different, and not being content with who they are. An incongruency between who we are and who we desire to be can create a lot of anxiety. So, how can you shift into the flow of healing this?

The mind is a very powerful tool. To work with your mind, you have to be friends with it. You don't have to like every thought it has, but you do have to accept your mind as is. Carl Jung, the father of analytical psychology, said we cannot change anything until we accept it. He also said that "neurosis is an inner cleavage—the state of being at war with oneself. Everything that accentuates this cleavage makes the patient worse, and everything that mitigates it tends to heal the patient."[1]

Let's break this down a bit. I talk about self-acceptance almost every day to the people I see because I see their tension, discomfort, anxiety, and their physical symptoms. I also see the light of their being, and the health within that is constant. The tug-of-war I see can happen between any of the dimensions of mind, body, and spirit. Often, there's tension between the ego and shadow aspects of self, what someone doesn't like about themselves and turns away from. The shadow is a normal part of the human experience, and it is where radical acceptance becomes so important.

Consider the various aspects of yourself like the facets of a gemstone. One facet is not better than another, and together, they create the unique whole that is you. When you call out all aspects of yourself, one by one, you reclaim the energy of the aspects you rejected. And as you shift your perspective, you allow these aspects to transform into something more useful for you in this moment.

For example, I used to describe some of my shadow parts as shy, hesitant, and emotional. Over time, I reclaimed those energies. I realized that part of my shyness was an aspect of my sensitive nature. I easily picked up on subtle energies and emotions. This also explains why I tended to be hesitant: I picked up so much information that it could overwhelm my decision-making abilities. I also saw that my being sensitive meant I felt things strongly, as anything could make me cry (even music videos). Over time, I've learned to look at all aspects of myself and embrace them. Once I grounded myself, I discovered my shadow parts have hidden strengths and gifts, such as helping me help others.

That's how things shifted for me.

The thing is, everyone has hidden strengths and gifts tucked away in the shadows. When we can welcome the shadow aspects, we see all of ourselves. It's not about liking what you see at first but loving yourself as you are. It's more than about loving yourself anyway; it's about loving yourself *any way* that you are. When you can acknowledge and hug in all of you, you will feel whole. You are already whole, but that tug-of-war inside keeps you from seeing yourself this way.

Confusion in the Body-Mind

I remember being nine years old, curled up in a ball in our living room. Nothing apparent was happening to me, but I was hyperventilating. That's what we used to call panic attacks back then—hyperventilating.

My parents didn't know what to do. They called my teacher. There was some minor confusion over an assignment. I don't even remember what I was upset about, but I still remember the overwhelming feeling that I didn't know what to do. My mind kept looping that thought, *I don't know what to do*. I couldn't think clearly, and my body reacted to my thoughts. My heart was racing, I was breathing too fast, and I felt jittery. I didn't realize then how powerful my thoughts were in creating my experience.

These days, we live in a world with a mishmash of information, and it's easy *not* to know what to do, with big and little things. Not knowing can easily throw people into anxiety or panic, which perpetuates confusion. Confusion can feel like chaos in the body. Energetically, it feels like static to me. Instead of a person's subtle energy field feeling nice and smooth, it feels like intense energy spitting out in all different directions without symmetry or order.

Remember the section in chapter 3 on reading your energy body? The energy field of confusion feels spikey or disorganized. The physiology will tend to match, too. The heart rate could be a bit faster, and the breathing more rapid and shallow. The upper half of the body could have more energy than the lower half, giving a person an ungrounded feeling. This is part of the mind-body disconnect.

So, what's the best way to deal with confusion? Acknowledge the "I don't know." If you're not sure how you feel, start with "I don't know." It sounds simple, but it means you have to pause with self-awareness to accept and love yourself in the confusion. Call it as it is. Say to yourself, *I don't know what to feel because [fill in the blank]*. When you first do this, there may be resistance. Although a part of you wants to know how you feel, another part doesn't. Recognize those opposing feelings and add a mindful aspect to the words going through your head. Again, calling out what is helps diffuse the intensity of the thoughts and feelings because you're no longer hiding from yourself.

Thought Patterns and Creation

Remember our discussion in chapter 4 about how thoughts become things? That holds true for positive and negative thoughts. So, even when we are *not* conscious of intense thoughts, it's still possible for them to manifest in physical reality.

One of my patients was going through post-partum anxiety and depression. Her body also ached, especially her left shoulder. During the osteopathic assessment and treatment, I told Alicia it felt like there was "a monster biting into her shoulder." She replied, "That's exactly what it feels like!" Alicia's shoulder pain represented what she felt but was resisting. The volume of one of her looping thoughts got turned up and subconsciously manifested its energy in the physical. She basically had a thought pattern stuck in her shoulder.

There are some other details to consider here. Recall from chapter 1 that the left side of the body represents the feminine. Alicia's pain was in her left shoulder. She was overwhelmed by her maternal responsibilities, and it felt like a monster biting into her shoulder. Do you see how the pieces start to fit together? I gave Alicia an osteopathic treatment, easing the tension and improving the flow of the fluids in her left shoulder. Together, we shined a metaphorical light on the monster, and we tended to the issue represented. She did this by using some of the exercises in this very chapter, including accepting where she was and acknowledging her different facets.

Understanding these stories helps because they are archetypal experiences everybody goes through. It's also natural for us to be able to flow through these experiences. We're better prepared to do that once we recognize how we feel and call it out.

Pressure—Letting Your Scream Out

When people are under pressure, I will notice a general restlessness in them. The pressure has been contained for so long it feels like a scream ready to explode. Most people aren't running around screaming, though, and that's a good thing. But the contained pressure needs to be expressed at some point.

One way is to literally scream—into a pillow, at the ocean, while watching a sports game. In doing so, you're give yourself permission to have "a tantrum" without destroying the world around you. In the 1970s, psychologist Arthur Janov studied screaming. He described it is a natural release for working through traumatic memories. His books *The Primal Scream* and *The New Primal Scream* explain the dynamics in depth. The primal scream is a phenomenon that has caught on in popular culture. During the pandemic, Iceland's tourism website allowed you to record your scream and then have it broadcast on a speaker into the Iceland wilderness.[2] It's a brilliant idea! The wilderness can handle the energy. The earth will hear you out and help you heal.

Another way to let your scream out is to imagine doing it. Your imagination of screaming—or yelping, whimpering, sobbing, or crying—will be the same (or very similar) to your brain as if you actually did it. I'll commonly ask patients to imagine themselves expressing an emotion with an imagined vocalization and movement to give it a safe outlet. Sometimes, I'll ask them to imagine themselves at the top of a mountain letting out a full-body scream. It's like letting a balloon deflate to release its pressure.

A third way to let any emotional pressure out is to *pick an animal that represents how you feel.* I'll use this for both kids and adults when they have difficulty choosing words to describe how they feel. We can release both the pressure to overanalyze as well as the emotional pressure at the same time. We are freeing ourselves to feel however we feel. Once you pick an animal that represents how you feel, you can then act out the animal (safely), imagine being the animal, draw the animal, or any other fun variation you can think of. These are such simple exercises that can have a profound impact. (See page 135 for additional ways to let your scream out.)

Steer Fear Toward Excitement

Just before her piano recital, my then-five-year-old daughter said, "Mommy, I'm scared and excited. You know what I mean?" This was her first piano recital. She had spent time preparing for it and was all big smiles, but she felt the butterflies, too. "Mommy, what if I mess up?" she asked me. "Then I'll feel bad for myself, or people will say, 'Oh, you messed up!' You know the piano recital is kind of a big deal." She had skipped out on a piano recital the year before, so these were not new feelings. But this was another year and another opportunity to deal with the same thoughts and feelings in a new way.

Does this kind of mental chatter feel familiar to you, too? Have you ever thought to yourself, *This is a big deal. What if I mess up?*

"Well, it is a big deal," I told my daughter, "but at the same time, it isn't. It's your first time, so it is exciting, but it isn't a big deal in another way because you can get through it. If you do it this time, you won't be as nervous the next time you have to do something where you get a chance to express yourself this way. That's a great thing." And then I added, "And if you do mess up, you'll still be your lovable, huggable self. Nothing will change that about you."

That's an important message for all of us, isn't it? We hold ourselves back because we're scared. But there's also excitement; after all, why else would we get the idea to do that very thing? Whether changing jobs, moving to a new place, making a new friend, or trying that new recipe, if we can step into the excitement of something we'd like to do even though we're scared, we will do so many more amazing things. It's okay to be scared. It's part of being human and a normal physiological phenomenon. In fact, the physiological sensations of fear are similar to excitement: the heart rate increases, breathing quickens, and muscles tense.

Remember the fight-or-flight response we discussed in Part 1? What we can do with fear is direct its physiology toward excitement. Please take a moment to review the section in chapter 3 on when to listen to fear and when to persist despite it. To shift your life experience, claim yourself as you! You don't have to fight fear and anxiety. It's a shift in your mindset that will help you. Notice your emotions and the physiological sensations accompanying them. Once you steer fear toward excitement, you can use that adrenaline to move in the direction you desire.

Adapting to Stress

Once you step into the excitement, you get to see how adaptable you are. Just because something is stressful doesn't mean you have to stay in a constant state of stress. The outer world does *not* have to determine your inner world. You can adapt to stress and do hard things in life.

Charlie Goldsmith is an energy healer from Australia who has been studied by physicians at hospitals affiliated with New York University. He shares this observation about our natural response to hearing something funny: The first time we hear a joke, we might laugh spontaneously. If we hear the same joke repeatedly, we might continue to laugh, but at some point, our laughter lessens. It's great to laugh, but it's not functional if we never stop. The same is true of our stress response. A stressful situation might trigger stress in the body, but we don't have to stay stressed because the body is adaptable. The difficulty comes when we avoid how we feel. We don't like to feel stressed, so we tend to resist it. A stressed person often tries to control their external world to avoid feeling stressed. The universe doesn't work this way, though. We can't shift the external world without shifting our internal world. The only way to change our experience of the world is to change the world within us. Peace must start from within.

This takes a conscious awareness of yourself, your thoughts, emotions, and behavior. You will start to notice a pattern in your responses, and it will take deliberate practice to choose *not* to run your neural networks' default patterns, not to take those heavily traveled highways. It also takes regular practice to establish new neural pathways. You change your neurochemistry and circuits with your mindset. Studies in neuroscience show that positive thoughts boost serotonin levels and create new nerve synapses, new connections, in the brain.

To *choose* new pathways, you must stay self-aware. Self-awareness is key to conscious manifestation. Without it, we default to our subconscious patterns for creation, and then it seems like life is happening to us. Either way, self-aware or not, we're always creating. It's just that there's a way to do it consciously.

How do you better access your innate rebalancing mechanisms? Be yourself. When you let yourself have your authentic experience, your mind-body-spirit comes into alignment. There is no right or wrong to our experience.

One way to become self-aware and let yourself be is with this Brain Dump exercise. It's a simple yet invaluable exercise. Here's what's involved:

1. Get your preferred writing materials and set a timer for twenty minutes—longer if you like.

2. Write what comes to you in a stream-of-consciousness brain dump. Write whatever thoughts bubble up into your awareness. Get them out from inside your mind and body.

3. When you're finished, give thanks, and get up to move your body for at least five minutes to assimilate the new space you created in your thinking.

We're all constantly growing and learning; that's part of the point of living. When you realize this, the challenging moments in life begin to take on new meaning.

A Growth Mindset Changes Everything

Switching from a fixed mindset to a growth mindset will make all the difference in your life. With a fixed mindset, we think our gifts and talents are set and can't change. So, let's say you don't score well on a test. With a fixed mindset, you will think you're not smart. But with a growth mindset, you will see this as an area where you can learn and grow. You don't interpret scoring poorly on the test as a verdict on how smart or worthwhile you are but as feedback on where there's room to learn.

I've had so many moments when I've been a perfectionist, and it kept me stuck. I couldn't move forward because I had to make things perfect before I could move on. The default with this mindset easily becomes not getting things done. Just the thought of the effort needed to achieve perfection can stop us in our tracks. Perfectionism can be understood as a fear of failure; it keeps us from moving forward. The good news is we can change this.

You can switch your thinking to a growth mindset that says, *Whether I fail or succeed, every moment is a growth opportunity.* This way of thinking eases the pressure to succeed. Instead of saying, "I don't want to mess up," you can say to yourself, "Oh! that happened. This is an amazing growth opportunity for me. What can I learn?"

Lindsey Stirling is a world-class violinist and dancer who combines the two in her performances. She was on television's *America's Got Talent* in 2010. When she didn't make it to the finals, the judges gave her specific notes for improvement. Lindsey accepted the feedback and kept at it. Now she tours the world performing for her fans.

Lindsey learned and grew. The challenges we face ask us to do the same. When things are difficult, there's remarkable potential to grow. We keep moving forward when we say, "I can learn," and when we ask, "What can I learn from this?" Whether you succeed or fail, it's a growth opportunity. Of course, if things go the way you'd like, it's easy to see you've learned something. But we also learn—and maybe more—from failure. When you feel you've failed, you have an opportunity to look at things differently, to widen your perspective and see how you can grow from the experience.

Helping vs. Controlling

Empathic and highly sensitive people tend to want to help others, which is beautiful. As your empathy and sensitivity grow, you'll find you need to conserve your energy and use it wisely. While we are meant to be social creatures who help each other, there's a balance to maintain. Compassion for others shouldn't be at the expense of your well-being.

There's also a line between helping others and controlling that is important to see. "Helping is the sunny side of control, " writes Anne Lamott.[3] Sensitive people also fall into the trap of people-pleasing to control a situation.

So, how can we tell the difference? Be aware of your reasons for helping. Are you trying to manage uncomfortable emotions, yours or the other person's? You can't control other people's feelings, but you can shift your own experience. Here are the questions I ask myself to help me see if I've lost sight of the fine line between helping and controlling. You may find these helpful:

1. **Why am I helping?**
   What is my motivation? Is it about my feelings and my need to fix or change the situation? Is my help welcome? Am I being asked for help? Am I helping out of expectation, my own or another's? Is it purely out of service, or am I looking to be rewarded?

2. **How does my choice affect me?**
   Do I lose myself or my values in agreeing to help? If my answer is yes, I reconsider my actions.

3. **Am I being considerate of myself and creating healthy boundaries?**
   In other words, can I be myself in the situation? When we're kind and sincere to ourselves, we're more likely to stay grounded and hold space with love and respect.

4. Am I resentful?

Feelings of resentment are a sign of overextending. This is when we need to pause and rebalance.

5. Am I being loving to myself?

Loving myself means being kind to myself and others. When I love myself, I don't need to put other people down to feel better about myself. I also care enough about myself to speak my truth and get out of harm's way. Another way to say this is to ask yourself if your compassion for others is balanced by self-compassion.

6. Am I being called to help?

Before I help someone, I ask myself, *Am I being called to help right now?* This is a huge learning experience. We can be supportive of someone without interfering in their growth process. A person is whole even when they are going through something uncomfortable. Trust the light in them and in yourself, and trust in the growth process. Sometimes, we are more helpful with a hands-off approach. Make sure you are being called to help before you intervene.

These questions can provide insight and reflect your state of being. Take your time as you develop more self-awareness.

Be-Do-Have

Be-Do-Have is a great way to remember the order of conscious manifestation. Often, we get trapped by the reverse order: Have-Do-Be. We think we have to *have* something (such as a piece of equipment) in order to *do* something (maybe finish a project), and then we will *be* happy. You can continue to carve out your life the Have-Do-Be way, but it's way less efficient and makes you work much harder.

Be-Do-Have is a path of much greater ease. It directs you first to be who you hope to be. Turn inward, and you will realize that peace and joy are within you, not outside of you. When you turn inward, you will feel the truth of your be-ing, and then, you'll be able to take steps to do whatever you dream of and ultimately have whatever you desire.

So, how can you *be* with more ease? Not by waiting for the big moments in life to save you but by appreciating all the little moments as they unfold. Enjoying the colors of the sky, the soft touch of a blanket, the miracle of your hands. Taking the time to meditate and consciously attune your vibration with the Oneness of life will allow you to go deeper still. It takes consistent practice to bring yourself into alignment and move from that place, but it's worth it!

When you find yourself rushing around, pause and appreciate where you are. Working on a project with an urgent deadline is much easier when I calm down and ground myself. I make it a priority to greet my kids and say hello to my family before I settle down to work on a project. Be-Do-Have is a great way to flow through life. Experiment with this approach and see what works for you.

How to Get Through Anything

The only way you can get through anything is moment by moment. Whether it's an easy moment or a difficult one, the present moment is all we have. Before I wrote this book, I read Anne Lamott's book *Bird by Bird*, where she tells a story about her brother having to write a school report on birds that he put off doing until the night before it was due. He was in a panic. Their dad told him all he had to do to find his way through was write that report bird by bird. I love that reminder.

Our bird by bird in daily living is our breath by breath. Each breath we take connects us to the next. There are moments in life of great emotional intensity when time seems to stand still, such as the death of a loved one or a divorce. The heavy emotions at these times might feel stifling and make it difficult to breathe. That's when you remember to take it breath by breath. You only have to be right where you are. In those moments especially, you need *you*, so keep breathing. You don't have to have everything figured out. Do whatever is called for in the moment, and be with yourself in each moment. This will help you see choices when you feel like you may have none. Your awareness can redirect your life.

Summary

An overactive mind is ungrounded and interferes with our intuition. To work with your mind, you have to be friends with it. A neutral and accepting presence is key to grounding the mind and accessing more fluid and clearer thoughts.

1. The ego mind wants to keep you safe in the box of what it knows.

2. You can only start where you are, even if that means acknowledging confusion or uncertainty.

3. Looping thoughts become thought patterns that can create physical manifestations.

4. Sometimes you need to let your scream out in a safe way.

5. Since the physiological responses to fear and excitement are similar, one way to work with fear is to steer it toward excitement.

6. Give yourself permission to fail. A growth mindset can change everything.

7. Be aware of the line between helping and controlling. There is no need to control or overhelp.

8. The key to conscious manifestation is first to be the love, peace, and joy that you are. Then you'll be in the flow of doing, and that doing will lead you to have what you desire. Remember that order: Be-Do-Have.

9. The only way to get through anything is moment by moment.

Now that you know more about grounding the mind, it's time to use the whole mind—the conscious and subconscious parts—like a compass to access your intuition and locate your true north.

CHAPTER 6

ACCESSING YOUR INTUITION

"You can access intuitive guidance when you let your thoughts flow and direct them toward your true north."

A patient I'll call Kathryn came to me distraught about a business situation. The business owner had died, and now unsettled matters and secrets were being revealed. Kathryn was in a frenzy trying to sort through it all without hurting anyone, and the stress was affecting her health. She couldn't focus or sleep because her mind was always racing, and she was gaining weight using food to soothe herself. When I saw her, I could hear the universe saying to her, *You're worried about nothing!* Kathryn's worries came from her assumptions about how people would take the news. She wasn't giving them a fair chance to respond but trying instead to manage everyone's responses.

Once she became aware of what she was doing, the big balloon of pressure deflated. She realized that the energy she was investing in control wasn't necessary, and as she shifted gears, her mind opened up to new possibilities. Her thinking flowed, and a path of greater ease presented itself. Her physical health also improved.

When the mind is grounded and aligned with the heart, we gain access to our internal compass. When we allow our thoughts to flow while mindful of them, the mind can navigate tough times.

Mindfulness and Butterfly Thoughts

Mindfulness is a nonjudgmental meta-awareness. A growing body of studies on mindfulness shows how beneficial it is. Mindfulness helps to improve sleep, alleviate stress and anxiety, strengthen the immune response, enhance cognition, and support relationships. It also improves our access to intuition.

A friend told me the idea of mindfulness sounded good, but she didn't know where to start. I suggested starting with what I call "butterfly thoughts," a helpful technique for beginners and seasoned practitioners of mindfulness. Here's how it works. As you notice your thoughts, you first say hello to them and let them flit like butterflies. Then, you imagine opening a window they can fly in and out of as they please. You don't have to catch any of these thoughts or push them away. A thought is simply a thought—you don't have to believe it. You can also feel a certain way, and it doesn't have to make sense. Understanding this will ease the intensity and flow of your thinking.

We typically want to catch the "good" or "positive" thoughts and push away the "bad" or "negative" thoughts, but this creates pressure and anxiety. When we try to hold on to happy thoughts, we can't fully breathe and be present with them, and when we try to contain negative thoughts, they can end up stuck somewhere in the body. But when we do nothing except notice our thoughts, those butterfly thoughts will naturally come and go in the movement that is life.

Mindfulness is about having a neutral awareness. You witness your thoughts as a kind, loving observer without judgment. The key here is nonresistance. Let your thoughts be free. Remember, just because you think something doesn't make it true, so you don't have to act on all your thoughts. You might also pick up on other people's thoughts if you're highly sensitive or empathic. Remain a neutral witness to all thoughts. The point of mindfulness is to be more fully present with your mind, body, and spirit.

So, say you're folding the laundry. You can do so with mindfulness. Instead of running through your to-do list or spacing out, let your senses take in the colors, textures, and temperature of the fabrics you're folding. Let your mind experience gratitude for the clothes you have, and let your heart open to the care you're giving yourself and those whose laundry you might also be doing. I've seen some of my patients take this concept into their personal and professional lives. First, they observe the thoughts, emotions, and behaviors in their personal lives.

Then, they observe their loved ones without judgment. And then they bring mindfulness to their work and other aspects of their lives.

My patient Jonah did this. He was anxious about giving presentations at work. However calm he might appear on the outside, Jonah felt all jittery inside. We talked about his being aware of his feelings without judging them. We also talked about having a growth mindset and allowing himself to fail. This wasn't an intention to fail but an acceptance to do what he could and let things unfold as they would. It took some time, practice, and becoming aware of his triggers, but bit by bit, Jonah shifted his thoughts and began to be more kind and loving toward himself. (The exercise called Finding Stillness in the Storm on page 137 helped him with this.) Jonah's increased self-awareness also helped him become more aware of his colleagues. He started to see that some of them were also nervous about presenting. Jonah hadn't noticed this before because he was distracted by his own anxiety. But now, he felt compassion for his co-workers and cultivated a more peaceful presence for them and himself.

New thoughts bring innovation. As Albert Einstein said, we cannot solve our problems with the same thinking that created them. Where do new thoughts come from? Our Higher Self—that part of you that is connected to the Oneness of all life. I suggest you practice freeing your butterfly thoughts for a few minutes several times a day and whenever your thinking is stuck. You'll start to develop a new way of thinking that's integrated with your intuition. This doesn't mean there won't be challenges. But when there are, you will have created a space where they can flow.

Your Why Is Your Compass

To keep your thoughts flowing while also directing them in a conscious direction, it helps to know your *why*. Why do you do what you do? What motivates you to do whatever you do? What is your deep why?

One of the immediate answers people give for the why of what they do is "to be happy." Everybody wants to be happy, but the key is not to externalize our happiness. If you find yourself saying, "If only [fill in the blank], then I would be happy," you're relying on external factors, which is not true happiness. Sensory pleasures and comforts can create feelings of happiness, but these are fleeting. They don't have roots. Physical comfort can be part of your why, but it's not the deep root of your why.

For your why to be a compass in your ideal life, you need a sense of greater purpose. This could feel like a calling, but it doesn't have to. Mainly, this is about attuning with the divine love within you, which desires to be expressed. You will never run out of love because the more love we share, the more we have. That's the wonderful paradox about love. Your deep why will be rooted in love. It will be about helping and serving others in some way. It doesn't matter what your job or profession is—any action done with love is an act of service, whether serving tea, planting flowers, showing up for a grieving friend, or helping clean up the ocean.

When you know your deep why, you are more likely to take the steps you need to take to keep going. Your deep why gives you a vision and momentum. As Henry David Thoreau wrote in *Walden*, "If one advances confidently in the direction of his dreams and endeavors to live the life which he has imagined, he will meet with success unexpected in common hours." Your deep why is your connection to your soul, which is love and light. When you follow your deeply felt why, your body, mind, and spirit align, and the universe meets that momentum in ways better than you can imagine.

I love seeing my patients get in touch with their deep why. It helps motivate them to take better care of themselves and heal from whatever difficulties they've been through. I see both the fear and the courage in their glistening eyes once they decide to understand themselves better. Their desire to love and serve makes the difficult steps of change worth taking, and stepping into love and service always brings them more happiness.

Keep Expanding Your Perspective

As you step into your deep why, your perspective on life shifts. To maintain your emerging optimism, keep expanding your perspective. Here you are reading this book, maybe in a room, maybe outdoors. The greater community is all around you, your country, the earth, the solar system, the universe, and so forth. You might know exactly what you are doing, but you can't predict the far-reaching effects of your actions. Still, somehow, they do matter. You matter.

When we're in a difficult situation, expanding our perspective can be challenging. We're so focused on the issue at hand that it's hard to see the larger context. The mind is powerful, though; if we harness its abilities, we can open up limitless potential. This takes a shift in thought.

It helps to do something to expand the connections in the brain and our view of what is possible. One easy way is to do something that isn't in your comfort zone or that is out of step with the usual. I'm not talking about anything dangerous but something as easy and silly as wearing your shirt backward. You could try writing with your non-dominant hand or walking backward for a bit. You might also literally look at things from different angles. Do a little something to help wake up different pathways in your brain. The cross-lateral movements we covered in Part 1 will also help do this. So will dancing organically. Kids are constantly shifting their perspectives as they play and tumble around. No wonder they are so creative!

It's also helpful to imagine things working out—even if it seems impossible. Audrey Hepburn would say, "Nothing is impossible. The word itself says, 'I'm possible!'" You don't need to know all at once how what seems impossible will be accomplished. Just start by clarifying the desire. Many people questioned whether my medical practice would work out, and sometimes, I wondered why they didn't have more confidence in me. Once, my dad asked me why I didn't just join a large health HMO. He said it would be so much easier on me. When I widened my perspective on my father's advice, I realized he cared deeply for me. He wanted me to do well and was afraid of the risk I was taking. I was afraid, too, but my vision was bigger than my fear.

I've seen many people recreate their lives after major transitions, such as divorce or the death of a loved one. At these times, there seem to be so many pieces to pick up. There's also a mourning period when everything seems heavy and flat. It's the messy time of the cocoon. Something beautiful can grow out of it, though. That's the silver lining—there's a transformation that makes going through hard things worthwhile. This view is a grander and more loving way to see life and the light in any situation. No matter how heavy things feel, there is light and purpose to all of this. We may not understand the why of circumstances or be able to see the big picture. Still, we can pause and remember that light exists and life is purposeful.

See the Ridiculousness in Things

Sometimes seeing the ridiculousness in heavy times is what's called for to lighten matters up. You know those times when you think, *Well, I could laugh or cry?* Sometimes, choose the laughter. Not in a way that bypasses your emotions. You still see the circumstances and how they could make you cry, but then you expand your perspective to see what is also funny or ridiculous about them.

I'd like to clarify why I chose the word *ridiculous* in this context. It's derived from the Latin word *ridiculus,* which means "laughable, funny, absurd," and from *ridere,* which means "to laugh." Something ridiculous can feel so comically absurd that it is nonsensical. When used in a positive way, the nonsensical aspects of what is ridiculous can be a stimulus for innovation because they break the boundaries of reality.

When you expand your perspective to see what is also funny or ridiculous about your circumstances, you might let yourself laugh *and* cry. We know that laughing is a great way to release tension and stress. Loving laughter can help guide us. It breaks through the heavy fog of thoughts and gives us moments of clarity. I often feel the universe laughing at us silly humans.

It's possible to find humor even in times of grief. At my dad's funeral, my brother and I saw a dear friend we hadn't seen in years. It can be so easy to slip back into the fun you used to have with old friends. I can't remember the conversation anymore, but we shared a moment of laughter—and it felt so good to laugh through our tears. My mom glared at us, understandably. But that shift in perspective with my brother and our friend lifted our hearts. When we can appreciate the ridiculousness that is part of life, we also notice that there is more love around than not.

The Vibrational Power of Words

The word *desire* stirs up different physiological sensations than the word *want*. *Want* is overused in our material-focused culture and sometimes falls flat. *Desire,* however, is a word that helps us access the well of potential that's always within us. It wakes up what yogis call the "kundalini energy," which runs midline from the base of the spine to the crown of the head and is the potential energy of creation within each of us. Desire creates momentum even before we take action. Stating what you desire is a clarity of intention that aligns your vibration with how you'd like your life to unfold even before it does. It's part of that Be-Do-Have dynamic we looked at in chapter 5.

It's amazing how different words create different vibrations that we can feel. The *authenticity* we feel when we say words is key to harnessing their power. Do you mean what you say? Can you feel it? This is why it might not feel the same when different people say the same words. When I'm teaching, students sometimes say, "It's interesting how you can get it when one person says it and not another." This could be a matter of resonance or timing, but I've also found that the vibration words carry are soulful and grounding when they're said sincerely. You can't fake this.

Table 11 on the next page summarizes what I feel when I say these different words sincerely. I invite you also to investigate what you feel when you say them. The words with an asterisk (*) are ones I've found have more potency and momentum. I believe this is so because they're words that originate from within us rather than outside. Of these, "I AM" is the ultimate statement of divine creation.

I had a patient with a lifelong history of allergic skin reactions. Jaime's skin improved dramatically after osteopathic treatment and some dietary and lifestyle changes. However, she still had the lingering mindset, "I am an allergic person." I had Jaime shift her "I am" statement to "I am at peace with myself and my environment." That change allowed her to exhale more completely, and she stepped into trusting herself even more.

Another patient was having fertility issues. Becca had already experienced huge shifts in her life. Part of Becca felt that maybe she didn't deserve to get pregnant, which created a wobble in her vibration, in how she was feeling. We worked on establishing a clear direction in her mind with the words, "My *dream* is to . . . my *hope* is to . . . and my *desire* is to . . ."

Table 11 - The Vibration of Words

Word	Vibrations
I desire*	Stirs up energy in the first chakra and wakes up the kundalini energy, a potential energy of creation.
I want	Felt in the gut, or the third chakra, where we are hungry for life and want to digest it. "I want" does not have the same energetic momentum as "I desire."
I hope*	Felt in the upper chakras—the third eye and crown chakras—where we receive inspiration from spirit. Hope is thought made divine (see chapter 9).
I dream*	Feels similar to "I hope." Think of Martin Luther King Jr.'s moving "I Have a Dream" speech.
I think	Mental energy that may or may not be connected to heart and spirit. "I think" doesn't have the same energetic momentum as "I hope" or "I dream."
I intend*	Intention has purpose behind it and activates the third and fourth chakras, or the solar plexus and heart.
I wish	Sends a message that is focused more on external happenings than internal shifts and doesn't imply accountability.
I trust*	Relaxes the lower chakras and connects them to the heart center, where we trust that the universe is abundant, that it does provide, and that all is well.
I believe*	Connects the heart with the throat chakra and third eye (the fourth, fifth, and sixth chakras). When we say, "I believe," we speak and think our heart's truth.
I love*	Opens the heart center, expands its field, and nourishes our whole being. "I love myself" is a beautiful message to send yourself daily.
I AM***	The ultimate statement of divine creation when body, mind, and spirit are aligned and all chakras are open. "I AM" is the most conscious way to be in the world: I AM love; I AM intuitive.

You can do this, too. Sit quietly and ask yourself: *What do I dream for my life? What do I hope for? What do I desire?* Meditate on each key word and see what comes up. The words *dream, hope,* and *desire* dig deeper within us than the words *want* and *wish,* which tend to be driven more by the external. How we think and speak affects our lives and ways of being. You can learn a lot about yourself from the words you use when talking to or about yourself. Also, the vibrations of words impact us whether we say them out loud or think them. Choosing your words wisely will also help you focus your energy. You'll find a helpful exercise, Finding Stillness in the Storm, that fosters a growth mindset on page 137. For now, let's continue to look closely at the power of words and mantras.

Where You Focus Grows

I used to love to complain. It felt so good to vent to a friend in the moment, but though that was true, complaining didn't make me feel better in the long run. In fact, the more I complained, the more there was to complain about. That's because where we place our focus grows. Once I understood this concept, I also made it a point to share it with my patients.

When we start to feel better, we experience what appear to be lots of little coincidences—"Hmm, I'm sleeping better, no longer have nightmares." "I'm breathing better." "I don't get as anxious." "My back hurts less." I call these coincidences "little miracles," and the more we notice them, the more we see them. This is also true for any perspective. It's your choice how you see something. This is not about a right or a wrong choice. In fact, you could acknowledge more than one perspective and be okay with them at the same time. You have the opportunity to grow with any perspective. But with a more conscious view, you can steer your life in a more positive direction. Priming the subconscious mind also helps us do this. Let's take a closer look.

Priming the Subconscious Mind

Your intuitive mind includes the vast subconscious mind, the part of the mind that is constantly working for us without our full awareness. The subconscious mind operates on autopilot; however, we can prime it to work for us in a conscious direction. We can point the subconscious mind toward our true north. Here are some ways to do that.

Use your mind as a search engine. As we discussed earlier, where we focus grows. Whatever we focus on also signals the subconscious to search for evidence that supports our thinking. So, to shift your subconscious search engine, you must also shift your focus. Use your conscious mind to pose various questions to your subconscious mind. You don't have to have the answers right away; they will be revealed to you in time. You can ask your subconscious anything, just as you would with an internet search engine. It's up to you to direct it. Here are some examples:

- How could I love myself more?
- How could I take better care of myself?
- How could I best serve others today?
- How can I grow through this?
- How could I have more fun in life?

I find these kinds of prompts helpful for people experiencing constant chitter-chatter in their heads. If your mind is constantly going, give it a specific job. Redirect it to work for you instead of against you. Let your mind become curious about healing and the nature of things.

Use mantras. A mantra is a word or phrase you repeat out loud or silently in meditation. In doing so, you consciously infuse your being with the vibration of the words. Choose a word or phrase that feels good and holds a high vibration. Here are some ideas:

I am love.

I am truth.

I am intuitive.

I am peace

I trust myself.

I accept myself.

I believe in myself.

I can learn.

You can also make a mantra more specific. For example, when I do yoga, I say to myself, *I am strong and flexible in body, mind, and spirit.* I breathe that statement into my whole being. It's amazing how it shifts my yoga practice. I feel an expansion in flexibility and strength without extra effort. I've tried it the other way, too, saying, *Ugh! I'm so inflexible,* and then that statement becomes a self-fulfilling prophecy. There are many ways to incorporate mantras into your life. These include:

Sit in meditation. You could sit quietly in meditation and say or think your mantra with each breath. If you'd like, you could use one mantra on the inhalation and another on the exhalation. For example, on the inhalation, you could say, *I trust myself,* and on the exhalation, *I let go of what no longer serves me.*

Meditate with mala beads. Buddhists and Hindus use mala beads, whether a bracelet or a necklace, to count each time a mantra is said. The mala adds a tactile component of movement to your mantra practice. Many cultures similarly use beads for prayer and contemplation. They have worry beads in Greece, and in the Catholic tradition, the rosary is used.

Move your body in meditation. You could add even more movement to your mantra practice by moving your body. In some yoga classes, for example, you pick a mantra to use during that day's practice. Another way is to say your mantra during a simple walking meditation.

Connecting with Your Future Self

Imagine your dream self of the future. Connecting with that version of you now will help fine-tune your compass and set your trajectory for true north. Any problems that arise can be solved by imagining that they will work out. Once you prime your mind this way, your vision and subconscious mind will get to work for you. You'll find you step into more synchronicity. You'll be in the right place at the right time.

You can also imagine that where you are right now is where you are meant to be in this moment. Where you are right now is a stepping stone toward what is in store for you. See if you can appreciate those stepping stones even when life feels hard. As you connect with your future self, it helps to be specific, but don't forget to keep the bigger picture in mind—that grand perspective of everything and who you are.

A patient of mine, Michelle, has been connecting with her future self for the benefit of both her family and herself. She spends much of her day caring for her five-year-old grandson, Tim, who is developmentally delayed and has learning difficulties. Despite the progress he's making, Michelle gets frustrated when Tim says "no" to an activity she or his teachers ask him to do. Michelle was at a loss. She wants Tim to learn and grow. We approached this situation in several ways, using multiple exercises in this book.

- *Cultivating a growth mindset (chapter 5, page 114) and adding a mantra (chapter 6, page 128).* Tim tended to say "no" to activities he wasn't as good at, such as handwriting. Even though Michelle knew he was smart enough and told Tim he was, he didn't feel smart when he wasn't good at something. Michelle and I chose the mantra "I can learn" for both her and Tim. Adding "yet" to the end of the statement "I can't do this" was another transformative bridge we built with the mantra: "I can't do that *yet!* But I can learn!"

- *Placing a hand on the heart (See the exercises Ways to Access Your Body's Wisdom in chapter 3, page 70, and Reading Your Heart in chapter 9, page 164).* To help Michelle trust herself, access her intuition, and connect with her grandson, we discussed how she could use her heart to read herself and her Tim. I told Michelle to place her hand on her heart and ask it questions. When something was true, she would feel an opening in her heart. She asked, "Is Tim mad at me? Is he upset with his teachers? Does he not get along with the other kids?" Michelle did not feel a heart opening in response to these questions because none of it rang true. But she felt her heart expand when she asked, "Is Tim afraid he's not good at it?" because *that's what he was feeling.* With this understanding, Michelle could take steps to help Tim learn.

- *Cross-lateral movements (chapter 1, page 22).* Tim showed signs of not always being able to cross the midline. For example, when anxious, he would wring his hands separately instead of together. He was also having trouble with fine motor control. We introduced cross-lateral movements to help him and Michelle integrate the left and right sides of the brain, which helps calm the mind, encourages fluid thinking, and improves coordination.

Michelle left our visit feeling empowered. Nothing had changed except her perspective and mindset. Now, she knows how to access her intuition, and with her help, Tim continues to make leaps and bounds.

Summary
You can access intuitive guidance when you let your thoughts flow and direct them toward your true north.

1. Let your thoughts flit about like butterflies. There's no need to hold on to good thoughts or push away bad ones. Non-resistance is key.
2. Know your deep why and let it ground you.
3. Keep expanding your perspective; it feeds optimism.
4. See the ridiculousness in a situation to help lighten your mind and flow with life.
5. Choose your words wisely. Whether you think them or say them aloud, words carry powerful vibrations. Use them to point your compass toward true north.
6. "I AM" is the ultimate statement of divine creation.
7. Be aware of the many miracles in daily life. Where you focus grows.

You can prime your subconscious to access more of your intuition and give yourself more momentum. Do this by using your mind as a search engine, making use of mantras, and visualizing your ideal future self.

There's Only Ever One Problem
Albert Einstein said we cannot solve a problem with the same thinking that created it. When some people first come to see me, they start by apologizing for their many problems and laundry list of concerns. They are pleasantly surprised when I tell them that there's only ever one problem: we're either in or out of balance with life. When we're out of balance, the more we look with that mindset, the more evidence

we'll find for being out of balance. For example, there is nothing wrong with factoring in the details about a medical condition you might have (lab results, etc.) Still, don't lose the forest for the trees, which means don't forget about the big picture. Let your symptoms be metaphorical messages for you. Let them have meaning. We all crave meaning. Appreciate all perspectives. If you're not making the kind of progress you'd like, consider how you're looking at things. Could you see them differently?

According to the spiritual curriculum in *A Course in Miracles*, the only problem we really have is thinking that we are separate and alone and forgetting that we are part of the Oneness that is all creation. When we can see this and consolidate our many problems into this one core problem, the solution is clear and certain. Ask yourself, *Can I remember that I am part of the Oneness? Can I think this and feel its truth in my body?* Once you believe and feel it, you know that this greater truth will resolve the particular problem upsetting you. I cannot say exactly how that resolution will unfold in physical reality because that is part of the miracle. In Part 3, we will explore this further as we dive into the intuition of spirit.

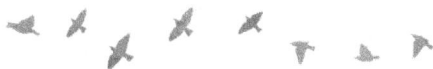

Exercises for the Intuitive Mind

Resetting Your Compass

I like to do this exercise first thing in the morning, as soon as I wake up, and at the end of the day. I review my thoughts and retract and transmute those I don't mean by using the intention/prayer I shared at the end of chapter 4. Resetting our compass helps us to

- Attune our thoughts to the Oneness of all creation
- Align our will with the Oneness
- Trust in something greater than ourselves

To do this, begin by reading the intention below to get familiar with it. Then, re-read each word with feeling, aligning mind, body, and spirit. Whether you think the words in your mind or say them out loud, feel the meaning of the words in your body. Let these ideas inspire your spirit. Here's how to set up:

- When waking, sit up in bed, propped up by pillows as needed.
- Place your hands comfortably in your lap or prayer position over your heart.
- Then, say or think the following words with feeling (or make up a variation to suit you):

    Dear Oneness (or God, Source, Universe, or any other term that speaks to you),

    I ask that
    my will be aligned with Your Will,
    my intention be attuned to Your Consciousness, and
    my thought be guided by Your Being.

    May I bathe in Your Light and Love, and
    may I let Your Light and Love

be a compass for
my thoughts, my words, and my actions.

May I feel this is every vibration of my being
and all throughout my day.

I trust in whatever way that my life unfolds,
and I know and feel there are miracles at every moment.

Thank you for being with me always.

A Mindful Walk

Take a mindful walk. You can do this anywhere—inside your home, around the neighborhood, in a park, or on a nature trail. Wherever you are, while walking, bring a neutral or loving presence to each moment. Mindfully check in with yourself as you walk. Be deliberate in noticing the following:

Each of your physical senses. What do you see? What do you hear? What do you smell? What do you taste? What do you feel in your body as you move through space? This noticing is similar to the body scan discussed in Part 1, except that now you're adding movement to the scan.

- How are you breathing?

- What do you feel emotionally? Where do you feel this in your body? Can you breathe into it?

- What are you thinking? Do any thought loops come up? Can you treat them like the butterfly thoughts we discussed in chapter 6?

- What do you connect with in your current environment?

- Optional: Add mindful photography to your mindful walk. This option was inspired by my friend and mindful photographer Marianne Ellis. Place your phone in airplane mode and notice what catches your eye while walking. Take photos of anything that calls out to you without troubling yourself over angles, lighting, or composition. At the end of your walk, see if your photographs have a theme.

Dropping Worries into the Well of Trust

Let's face it: worries creep in because we're human, and our worries can turn meta if we start to worry about our worries. Ahh! The mind needs something to do, a job to keep it occupied, so we might as well give the mind something more productive to do. Try this:

1. Imagine that you are dropping your worries into a deep well—a deep well of trust. (I love this visual!)

2. Add movement to this visualization by using your hand to pretend it's drawing a worry out from wherever you feel it in your body. If you're unsure where this worry is in your body, pull it out of your head.

3. Then, drop the worry into the deep well. You can also pretend that the well transmutes worries into light. It doesn't matter how many worries you cast into this deep well of trust because the well is infinite.

When we add movement to visualization, it gives your imagination more impact—the way dancing helps with personal expression. When your hand picks the worry up, that's acknowledgment, and then by putting it into the well, the movement emphasizes your choice to pivot, let go of the worry, and sink into trust with it. You start to clear the clutter of the mind and make a more comfortable home for your being. It's powerful imagery!

Three More Ways to Let Your Scream Out

In addition to the exercises on page 110 for Letting Your Scream Out, here are three more ways to help you let built-up pressure out.

Scribble Art

I originally made up this exercise for an eight-year-old boy who was angry for good reasons: he couldn't be around other kids because he had a serious chronic illness that affected his immune system—and then the pandemic hit. He became so angry he just wanted to throw things, and throw them he did! He broke an iPad. His parents were at a loss. I told the boy and his parents: "Emotions can be intense. Scream them out with crayons. Get a box of cheap or almost used-up crayons, and scribble your anger out onto paper until the crayons break." The permission to break something can be so freeing, so if you need to, keep it safe. This exercise is sometimes more challenging for adults to do than kids.

Splatter Paint

If you've got the space to make a mess, splattering paint to release your emotions is a fun option. Splatter paint studios and rooms have become popular and are popping up in various areas.

Rip Up the Recycling

Another way to express your scream is to give yourself permission to rip up something and throw it out. Rip up the cardboard and throw it back into the recycling bin. Stomp on the bubble wrap. If this starts to feel like fun, that's the point. You *can* express yourself in safe ways.

Make Your Mark

Peter Reynolds's children's book *The Dot* has inspired people all over the world. It's about a girl in an art class who doesn't think she's any good at art. At the end of the class, she still has a blank canvas. The teacher tells her simply to leave her mark. So she does, by literally marking a dot on the paper. Then the teacher says to her, "Now sign it." The next day, the girl is amazed to find that the teacher placed her work on the wall. It was too easy. It was just a dot. So she decides to make another dot, an even better dot. She goes on to make many dots and circles, and a whole collection emerges. Another kid looks at the dots and says, "Wow, I could never do that." And the cycle starts again. Make your mark. Yes, you can.

We can do this in the world: make a mark that is uniquely ours. There isn't any trying because you can't be anyone else but you. You're the best and only you there is! That makes you so precious. It also means there's no competition because no one can be you but you. Nor can you be someone else. But we can all inspire one another with the unique and loving expressions that are our gifts to share.

Try this exercise to drive this truth home inside yourself:

1. Draw a circle.

2. Fill the circle with whatever color(s) you desire. Let it represent how you feel in the moment. Don't put much thought

into it. You could color the whole circle or just parts of it, and you decide when it's done. There's no right or wrong.

3. Sign it.

Doing this exercise regularly would make a great art journal.

Finding Stillness in the Storm

When life gets chaotic, you don't have to get swept away by it. Consider the situation from the eyes of Love. Using mindful statements like the ones I share here can help you see challenges with a loving awareness; they help you reframe your perspective.

Table 12 - Mindful Statements:
    Moving from a Fixed Mindset to a Growth Mindset

FIXED MINDSET	GROWTH MINDSET	DESCRIPTION
"Oh no!"	"That's interesting!"	Difficulties are stepping stones for soul growth when supported by the stance, "That's interesting! I wonder what magnificent shifts are in store for me."
"I can't believe that happened."	"That happened. I feel (whatever you feel), and it's okay to feel what I feel."	Instead of staying in a frozen state of disbelief, step into the momentum of acceptance and the next steps.
"I can't believe they did that."	"People do cruel or horrible things when their soul is not grounded in the heart center."	People are capable of terrible things when subconscious trauma patterns of fight, flight, or freeze drive them like programmed robots.
"Everything is out of control."	"I want to be in control, but I can't be in total control. I trust in something greater directing life."	Maybe things feel slippery or out of control—but it's an illusion that we have total control in the first place.

Table 12 - Mindful Statements *(continued)*

FIXED MINDSET	GROWTH MINDSET	DESCRIPTION
"I messed up."	"That didn't work out as planned, but I am always learning."	Instead of focusing on a failure, shift your perspective to see how you can grow from the outcome.
"I'm too tired to get anything done."	"I choose to prioritize self-care and rest right now."	Sometimes, you need to take a break to rest and reset.
"I'll never figure it out."	"When life is chaotic, I focus on what I can do now."	When life is chaotic, take it moment by moment. Keep breathing. Whatever you can do at this moment is enough.
"I don't know what to do."	"I can move through this breath by breath."	You can provide a loving presence for yourself in difficult times moment by moment.
"I don't know what to think" or "I can't stop thinking about it."	"I can open a tiny door in my mind."	When you feel stuck or unsure, sometimes all you need is to open a tiny door in your thinking to give your mind space and permission to be.
"There are so many decisions to make."	"I get to choose my adventure."	Think of life as a "choose your own adventure" book, full of trials, twists and turns, and opportunities to choose how you will proceed.
"Everything is so hard."	"I trust the life process, and I can do hard things."	When life is messy, remember the butterfly. The pupa stage of the butterfly is also messy; it's also transformative.
"This will never end."	"A constant in life is change. This too shall pass."	Challenging times can feel endless, but they aren't. The seasons constantly change.

Realize there's something grander at work in all of life, and understand that you never have total control. When you experience a life storm, remember there is a stillness at the storm's center. You can witness the chaos and remain at peace from this potency within you at the center of any storm. Breathe in the stillness. Breathe in the stillness. Being in that stillness, the calm eye at the storm's center, you can expand the stillness, which will help dissipate the storm.

Talk to Yourself Like Your Own Best Friend

When I don't know which direction to go, I pause and then start a conversation with myself. I include Spirit in these conversations (more on this in Part 3). I always ask for help because it's much easier that way. I have a meta-conversation with myself as if I were my best friend or parent, someone who wants to support and encourage me.

You can have this kind of loving conversation with your mind, too. Throughout the day, talk to yourself as you would to a dear friend. Would you say those thoughts to a friend? Would a friend hang around if you kept talking like that? If not, then retract and transmute those thoughts and start anew. Sometimes, you may have to be strict with your mind to remind it to play nice!

A Photo of Your Younger Self

This is one of my favorite exercises for tapping into more love for ourselves.

1. Find a favorite photo of yourself when you were little. Aw! look at you as a little munchkin. Aren't you so adorable and lovable? If you don't have a photo of yourself as a child, choose any other favorite photo of yourself.

2. Place the photo where you will regularly see it, such as near your bathroom sink or mirror.

3. Whenever you see this photo of yourself, send love to that person. If your photo is next to your bathroom sink, you can easily do this every morning and night when you brush your teeth.

When you send love to the person in the photo, you are sending love to yourself. Self-love is essential for healing. As my friend Maudy Fowler says, "You are here for love, by love, to love."

Conversations with Younger Selves

Everyone desires to be seen and heard at every stage of life. When we don't feel seen and heard, we don't feel balanced and whole. Your mind is constantly seeking. When we go within to have a conversation with ourselves at different stages, we allow ourselves to heal the past hurts that still affect us today. Here's how you can do this:

- Think of a time that still makes you cringe. Don't pick anything traumatic unless you feel safe facing this alone.

- Let your younger self express everything it needs to—the good, the bad, the ugly—without holding back.

- Then, let your present-day self respond to your younger self in whatever way feels like a gentle, loving embrace. Be sure to end with some kind of loving appreciation.

This is a great exercise to combine with "A Photo of Your Younger Self" and the "Emotional Freedom Technique."

Small Steps Done Consistently Create Extraordinary Results

Let me repeat that: small steps done consistently create extraordinary results. Consistency is the key. There's now a whole science behind forming new habits. Here are some key tips:

1. **Be mindful of your big picture WHY** (see chapter 6).
   Be consistently mindful of what you hope to do and WHY you desire to do it. You'll feel amazing if you incorporate this new routine into your life. Whether it's a simple breathing exercise, healthier eating habits, or doing something fun daily, healthy habits fuel our love for life with vibrancy, happiness, and peace. Can you imagine it? Soak up these feelings now to give you the momentum you need.

2. **Schedule it.**
   Self-care is _not_ a luxury. It's a necessity. Prioritize your time to include your healthy habits.

3. **Reward yourself.**
   You know the saying, "It's not just about the goal but the journey"? Be specific about what you'd like to accomplish and reward yourself along the way. Maybe if you meditate seven days in a row, you'll treat yourself to a new book, and after 21

days, you'll treat yourself to a spa. (Oh! The thought of a trip to the spa—more self-care—can be so motivating for me!)

4. Be your own cheerleader.
Whether you make a basket or stumble, be ready to cheer yourself on. Maintain the belief that you can do it. Assume you'll be consistent rather than thinking you're doomed to fail. If you fall, brush yourself off, remember your WHY, and get back to it. Yes, you can do this!

5. Have an accountability buddy.
Is there a friend, family member, or colleague who would like to develop a habit, too? You can regularly check in with each other and encourage each other.

Go ahead and get excited! Let those feel-good emotions propel you forward. You are your own why.

Emotional Freedom Technique: Tapping

The following tapping basics are adapted from Gary Craig's Emotional Freedom Technique (EFT), which you'll find at emofree.com. EFT, also known as "tapping," is an easy-to-learn, self-help tool using acupressure points to help you ground and recenter yourself. When you feel stuck because of a particular thought loop, emotion, or even physical symptom, EFT can help you move through the stuckness.

1. **Choose** the thought you'd like to work on. Be specific. Here are some examples:

   I'm so overwhelmed with (whatever that might be for you).

   I am frustrated about (whatever you're frustrated about).

   I'm tired of (whatever this might be for you).

2. **Notice** where you most feel this thought in your body—it could be in your shoulder, abdomen, back, neck, etc.

3. **Check the intensity** your emotional or physical discomfort on a scale of 0 to 10, with 0 being no discomfort and 10 being the most discomfort. If you prefer a visual, you could use the scale "happy face" for no discomfort and "very sad face" for the most discomfort.

Figure 6 - Scoring the Intensity of Discomfort

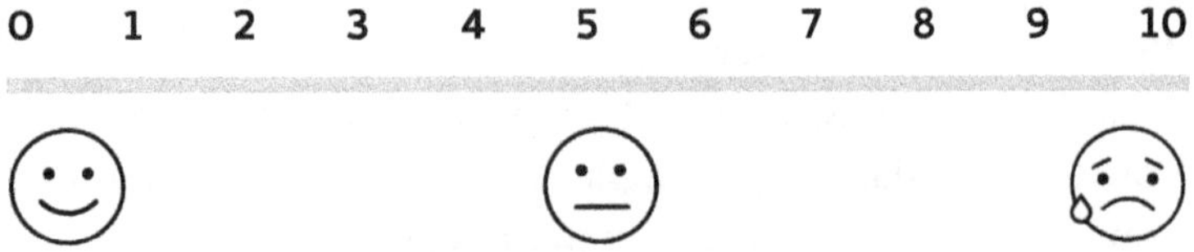

0   1   2   3   4   5   6   7   8   9   10

4. **Create** the **setup statement(s)** you will say three times while tapping. You can use the same statement or mix it up to address variations of the problem. The setup statements are meant to both **acknowledge** the problem **and accept** yourself anyway.

Even though I (acknowledgement of discomfort, whether a physical symptom or mental-emotional thought-feeling), I deeply and completely love and accept myself.

Examples:

Even though I have this dull headache, I deeply and completely love and accept myself.

Even though I'm so nervous about this interview, I deeply and completely love and accept myself.

5. **Tap first on the karate chop point** of one hand while saying your setup statement(s) three times.

Figure 7 - Karate Chop Point

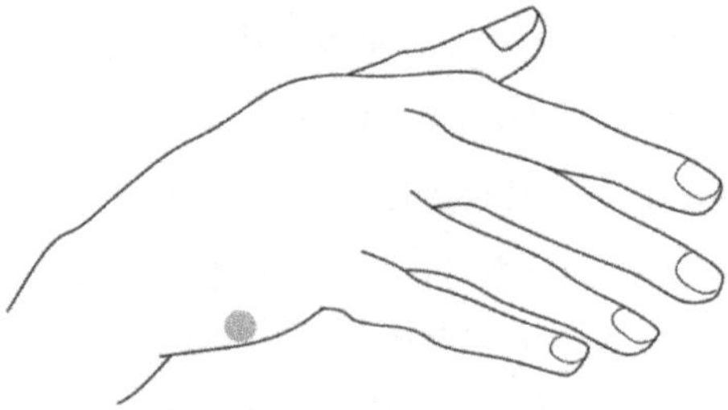

6. **Continue with the tapping sequence** illustrated below while saying your setup statements(s) three times at each point. After the karate chop point, move on to the inner eyebrows,

then the side of the eyes, under the eyes, under the nose, under the lip, under the collarbones, under the arms (level to the nipple in males and to the bra strap in females), and end at the top of the head.

Figure 8 - EFT Tapping Points

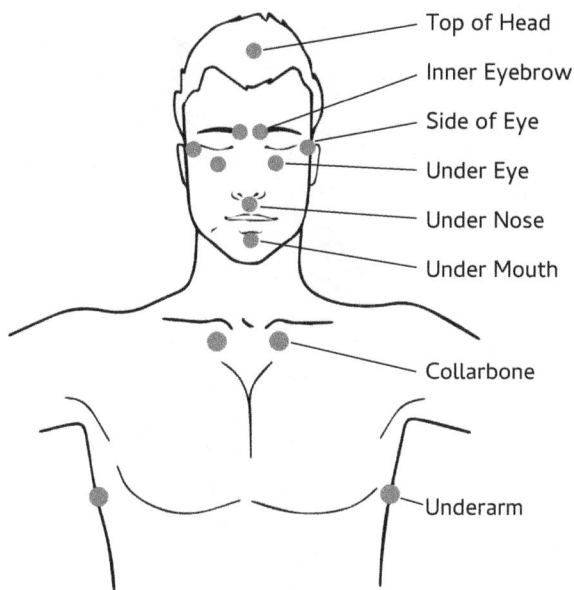

7. **Take a deep breath**. When you finish tapping at all points, check in and re-evaluate your discomfort on a scale of 0 to 10. If it is still high or has even increased because of the issues brought up, repeat the following phrase at each point:

Even though I still have (state the problem), I deeply love and completely accept myself.

Keep tapping until your discomfort level is 0 or as low as possible. Be persistent!

Tap for any problem, big or small, and see yourself transform!

PART III

The Intuitive Spirit

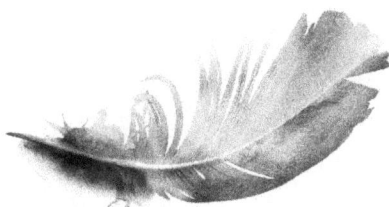

First, it's important to note that spirituality is not the same as religion. Religions are human-made constructs that can evolve (or devolve) with the people involved. Every religion has both helped and hurt humanity in some way. At its highest integrity, religion can enhance a person's connection to Spirit and provide comfort and guidance. However, religion does not determine your spirituality. This book makes no assumptions about your affiliation to any religious organization. Everyone is welcome.

We are all spiritual beings. There's no getting around that. To be human is to have a body, mind, and spirit. For our discussion about the intuitive spirit, I will use the terms *Oneness, Universe,* and *Spirit* to represent the Source that creates and connects all life in some miraculous way. You can replace my words with the term that resonates for you, whether God, Allah, Jehovah, Elohim, Universal Consciousness, Life Essence, Sacred Essence, Source, Creator, the Divine, Our Maker,

Higher Power, the Stillness, etc. Although there are not enough words to describe Spirit fully, we will still enjoy rich conversations about the infinite Spirit.

Once more, there are exercises throughout the chapters ahead to help you experience the information shared. Practicing the exercises will help bring this book to life for you. Practice the exercises that call to you—you don't have to do them all. With that, I look forward to exploring the intuitive Spirit with you.

CHAPTER 7

SPIRITUAL BEINGS HAVING A HUMAN EXPERIENCE

"As spiritual beings, we are expansive light and love with infinite potential. We are here to have a human experience, which includes sadness and grief and joy and happiness."

When my oldest was five, she asked me, "Mommy, does outer space ever end?" I answered her honestly: "I don't know." I could have come up with something because I have plenty of opinions, but I had nothing solid to go by. She followed up with another question: "Mommy, if God created the universe, who created God?" Well, that will have to be a never-ending mystery, I explained to her. Our minds aren't equipped for that understanding.

Later, when my youngest was five, I turned the table and asked her questions. "Where did you come from?" She answered, "From you, Mommy!" I persisted, "But where did you come from before then?" She said, "From heaven, of course!" "What's it like in heaven?" I asked her. She gave me a funny look: "I don't know! You came from heaven, too!"

That one statement fills me with warm fuzzies: "You came from heaven, too!" Those warm fuzzies can shape my days. What about you? What would it feel like to constantly remember you are divinely created, part of the universal oneness that in its essence is pure light and love? Would your day feel any different? See how it feels to you to say one of these "I AM" statements:

"I AM divinely created."

"I AM part of the Oneness."

"I AM pure light and love."

Do you feel it? What would shift in your life if you believed this and could feel it?

"We are not human beings having a spiritual experience. We are spiritual beings having a human experience" are the well-known words of French philosopher Pierre Teilhard de Chardin. I wonder what he felt and saw when writing those words. Even though we can't always see it, we are beings filled with light and love.

In truth, 97 percent of our mass is made up of the same elements that make up stardust—CHNOPS, which stands for Carbon, Hydrogen, Nitrogen, Oxygen, Phosphorus, and Sulfur, also known as the building blocks of life.

I think about all this often—like when I'm having a difficult day or feeling hangry, when the house is a mess, when I'm dancing with my kid, splashing in the pool, or enjoying a delicious meal. As spiritual beings, we are expansive light and love with infinite potential. We are here to have a human experience, which includes sadness and grief and joy and happiness.

Soul and Spirit

Every person has a soul, which is a unique expression of Spirit. Is the soul the same as Spirit? Yes and no. Spirit is the expansive oneness from which all things emanate. Your soul is a part of the vastness of Spirit connecting everything. In other words, Spirit is the source of all that is, including your soul, which is an emanation or expression of Spirit. The terms "your spirit" and "your soul" can be used interchangeably with the understanding that your soul is part of the human being that is itself part of Spirit. I use "s" when I mean your spark of spirit to distinguish it from the all-encompassing Spirit.

International speaker and author Anita Moorjani uses a beautiful analogy to distinguish soul and Spirit. She experienced a near-death experience that deepened her understanding of life and then returned healed from the metastatic breast cancer that brought her to death's door. Her doctors were perplexed. Anita wrote about her experience in beautiful detail in her book *Dying to Be Me*. She writes that each soul is like a finger on a hand and that all individual souls are connected. During our human experience, it's not always apparent that we're part of the same hand. We tend to see only the fingers that look separate from one another, making it easy to fight, argue, and compete. Anita's near-death experience gave her the grand realization that we are individual souls emanating from one universal Spirit. Each *soul* is precious and needed for its unique expression. No soul can fill another's role.

Our souls remember that we are all connected, but the individual's ego mind has forgotten. As we discussed in Part 2, ego thoughts tend to be loud, distracting us from our intuition, our inner knowing. Listening to the whispers of guidance that come to us from the soul takes conscious awareness. The soul's intuition and guidance come from Spirit. The word *inspire* means "to breathe in spirit." A spark of inspiration is the light of Spirit shining through. Spirit is also the source of your body's intuition—after all, your body is the human home for your spirit. You'll feel this when body, mind, and spirit are aligned and grounded.

Near-Death Experiences

I am thankful to know multiple people who have had a near-death experience (NDE for short) and shared their experiences with me. During an NDE, the soul disconnects or loosens its connection from the body. The trinity of the body, mind, and spirit are split and no longer aligned. After the NDE, there can be a dichotomy between what the soul consciously remembers and what the body remembers. Basically, the soul had one experience while the body had another.

In a couple of the NDE stories I've heard, the soul's experience during the NDE was blissful, sometimes seeing angelic beings and a spectacular loving light. On the Earth plane, however, the body experienced something else entirely, such as obnoxious sounds, physical pain, and panic. While the soul was in a blissful out-of-body state, the body was left in crisis on the operating table. When the soul returns to the body, it becomes aware of the body's pain and trauma. The mind is also in a state of shock, trying to sort out and connect the magnificence of the NDE with the body's pain.

Two people told me they didn't feel like themselves for a long time after their NDEs—months for one and years for the other. Despite the soul's joyful experience, they were left in a heightened state of anxiety they didn't have prior. I've seen patients experience a similar kind of shock from major surgery. In those cases, they didn't remember the situation, while those who've had NDEs do. For example, Dan came to me like that. He had cardiac bypass surgery and never felt the same since. He was stuck in an anxious fight-or-flight state that wasn't his norm. Dan didn't remember anything going awry during the surgery, but the surgery was still a shock to his body.

In all these situations, I suggested the person let the soul and body have a conversation (similar to the conversation with your body described in Part 1). To feel whole, the body needs to know what the soul went through, and the soul needs to know what the body went through. I also incorporate somatic trauma release work to help them, whether cranial osteopathy or therapeutic exercises. This integrative approach helps them return to a more balanced state of being. NDE stories are a perfect example of how we are spiritual beings having a human experience.

The Infinite Trust Fall

Deep down, we all know we are beautiful beings worthy of love— every one of us, regardless of what we've experienced. The hard part is expanding or bringing this knowing from our spirit to mind and body. Perhaps you read the first sentence of this paragraph and felt your mind push back on the statement. This is an example of the mind as a conflict creator. It's one thing to say, "I am worthy of love," and another to feel that deeply in your cells.

Being able to feel your worthiness requires a deep trust in the Universe. It can feel like an infinite trust fall. The conventional trust fall is a team-building exercise where one person falls backward and trusts that the other person will catch them. My version of the trust fall asks you to fall into the infinite loving arms of Spirit. It goes like this:

1. Imagine putting all your trust in the Universe, the Oneness.

2. Then inhale deeply and sigh all your worries out.

3. Lay down and relax your muscles one by one. Let yourself sink into the surface you're lying on. Let go completely, as if you were falling yet trusting you will be caught by the hands of the Universe. There's no need to hold on. Let go until you feel weightless because the hands of infinite light and love now hold you.

4. You can place everything in these hands—your hopes, dreams, and worries. See if you can imagine and feel an infinite trust in every part of your being. See how far you can allow yourself to let go. The Universe will guide you.

Enlightened and Still Human

No matter how enlightened you may become, you're still a human being. You will still have human experiences. You've still got to get out of bed in the morning, go to the bathroom, brush your teeth, cook, eat, clean up, and all the rest of human living. You've still got to interact with other people and the world. Some people might get on your nerves, and though you try to be patient, you'll know when it isn't happening because you won't feel quite right. Body, mind, and spirit won't be aligned. So, what I'm saying is, take it easy on yourself.

More conscious people tend to get down on themselves because they feel they "should" be able to handle difficulty better. The ego sneaks this comparison game into your consciousness regardless of how conscious you are. As you become more aware, let yourself lighten up. Some days will go more smoothly than others, and though your ego will try its ways of protecting you, you can't always skip over difficult feelings. You also can't use spirit to bypass difficult emotions. Even though you are light and love in essence, you will still experience challenges. Let yourself be.

I remember once feeling embarrassed by my behavior. I said some things that were not taken the way I meant them. A part of me knew there was nothing to be embarrassed about, that my embarrassment was my ego's concern about someone else's thoughts about me. I could have said to myself, *You shouldn't be embarrassed. Get a grip!* But I couldn't. It wasn't how I felt. I gave myself some time to feel through it and process it. I hugged a tree, and I emerged through it. We are all still human beings with egos, so be compassionate to yourself, whatever you are going through.

Embrace Your Humanness

Even when we understand the greater spiritual perspective, we still have visceral human responses. They may feel like opposing truths, but we can honor both because we are multidimensional beings. To ignore or push away a part of our experience would be inauthentic. Your spirit is embodied here on earth to understand what it is like to experience a rainbow of emotions and circumstances. Your mind may tell you that you must feel grateful for what you have, but you can be scared about finances at the same time. You're allowed to feel more than one way. You can be thankful and afraid. Some suffering is inevitable as we grow. After all, we have to face our fears to discover what we're capable of.

Though some emotions may feel more positive, there's really no good or bad in the human experience in terms of how lovable you are. Babies, toddlers, and little kids instinctively know this and flow from one emotion to another while still completely in love with themselves. In mere seconds, they may be thrilled with you, angry, and forgiving. They have no resistance to their being and fully accept themselves at every moment. No wonder they are so creative and loving! Of course, we don't aspire to be adult toddlers; instead, the hope is that through the years, we will become more aware of our impact on the world and behave with more conscious intention as we flow through our emotions with love and ease.

Embrace all of you, and you may be surprised by the comfort and peace you can give yourself. Embrace your sadness and grief; they show you love and care. Things will change; they always do. Embrace your happiness and joy; they also offer you love and care. When you embrace all of you, no matter what, you realize you are always whole. When we feel whole, we do not need to hurt others to feel better. Love yourself through all of it. Love yourself any way you are. You are a spiritual being having a human experience.

Be curious about your experiences, even the uncomfortable ones. For example, if you feel sad, walk yourself through it. What is this amazing feeling of sadness? It is an honor and privilege for our souls to feel all of human life. Imagine if you didn't know the pleasure of eating a delicious meal, the delight in learning how to ride a bike, or the lump in the throat when saying goodbye to a loved one. In pure spirit form, you wouldn't be able to know what those experiences feel like in the mind and body. There's beauty in the ups and downs of the human life. As humans, we get to experience our stories through multisensory input while getting to know our souls and exploring our infinite potential.

Growing Without Suffering

We can grow without suffering, but it requires conscious effort. We must first wake up to the truth that we are divinely created and part of the Oneness. Humans are on a never-ending quest to discover who we are, where we came from, and where we are going—the mystery that gives life so much meaning.

In the Disney Pixar movie *Soul*, they tell the story of the young fish who says to the older fish, "I want to see the ocean. Where's the ocean?" The older fish answers, "Well, you're in it. It's everywhere." The younger fish replies, "No, that's just water." The older fish smiles at this because it knows that what the younger fish is looking for is right there and everywhere. The younger fish is surrounded by the ocean it seeks.

What we are looking for is already with us, too, because we are part of the Oneness. Our souls are always home; we are never separate from the Oneness. We think what we want is somewhere outside of us to be found. But when we persist in looking outside ourselves, we block ourselves from seeing that we already have what we seek—we are already home. When we pause, go inward, and rest in the stillness, the world outside us starts to look different. As you recognize the light of your soul, you will begin to see the world in a different light. You will start to see the Oneness of all life and the true reflection of your inner and outer worlds. The "ocean" is in you and around you.

We are co-creators of our lives, but it takes conscious self-realization to see this. Stepping into your role as a co-creator is about making conscious choices and taking conscious action. Sometimes, you'll feel like a passive passenger on your life journey. Remind yourself who you are: a co-creator. You get to make choices. You get to create. You get to be an active part of your life. Accepting this will propel you forward. Can you wake up and accept who you truly are? Can you accept that your earthly existence is also a spiritual one? That you are a co-creator? That every experience is guiding you to grow?

It's as if we are living a crazy experiment to explore the question, "What if we were separate from the Oneness?" This experiment has us figuring out how to get back to the Oneness when the truth is we are already and still a part of it, despite our egos' attempts to convince us otherwise.

Intention, Love, and the Embodiment of Soul Consciousness

What's the difference between intention and consciousness? These concepts are so vast that they are worth revisiting. Let's review my working definitions of intention and consciousness from chapter 4. Intention is purposeful thought, which is a feeling-thinking vector needed to express love. Consciousness is awareness of the soul, which *is* love. I use the terms *consciousness* and *love* interchangeably. When I say consciousness, I'm also referring to soul consciousness.

Now let's take that a bit further. In addition to Love, there is *Light*. Light is Divine guidance—Divine wisdom, Divine information, Divine knowing, Divine Truth, and Divine understanding. Love and Light are intertwined and cannot be separated. Love and Light are eternally part of the soul and Spirit. If we describe Love as *the awareness of the soul (and Spirit)*, then Light is *the wisdom of the soul (and Spirit)*. When intention is directed by Divine guidance, the intention carries the brilliance of the Light. Intention on its own is not alive. I think of the difference between turning a light bulb on in a room versus sunlight. There's something different about them, and it's more than the wattage and wavelengths. The sun feels alive! Similarly, a person moving through the world with soul consciousness has that spark of life. You can see the light *and* love in the brightness of their eyes. The light of your soul—your *inner* light—is also a *loving* light, a *divine* light.

Intention needs soul consciousness—a consciousness of the divine light within—to come alive. Being aware of our thoughts without being aware of the light of our souls is not fully living. We need both intention and soul consciousness to create. Intention without love is robotic and often destructive. We see this in the world's violence and wars. Intention without love does not sustain life. Loving intention creates the peace necessary for life and springs from the realization that we are all part of the Oneness of Creation. To reiterate: Intention + Love = Creation. We cannot create without love. It is love that sprang forth from the void of the Oneness and led to the creation of the universe.

Being human is an incredible opportunity to embody our own soul consciousness. A loving intention infuses into the electromagnetic field of the heart and throughout our whole energy field, body, and brain. Life comes from Spirit. When we are aware of the love of our soul—our true nature—then body, mind, and spirit align, and we can fully experience life. We can feel love, see love, hear love, think love, and act with love. In essence, we can be love because we realize we already are love.

The Fibonacci Sequence and Surfing the Waves

It is in our nature to blossom. Interestingly, mathematics has shown this to be so in the Fibonacci sequence and the golden ratio. The Fibonacci sequence is a series of numbers in which each number that follows in a sequence is the sum of the two numbers preceding it. For example, if we start with 0 and 1, the Fibonacci sequence would be as follows:

0, 1, 1, 2, 3, 5, 8, 13, 21, 34 . . .

As the sequence continues, each number is approximately 1.618 times greater than the preceding number. The further the sequence goes, the closer it gets to this golden ratio.

You can think of the golden ratio as representing your true nature. The golden ratio shows up throughout nature—in spirals, ferns, and the development of the fetus and the brain. All nature has to do is be herself, and she will be an ever-closer expression of the golden ratio.

If you were to graph the Fibonacci sequence in terms of its approximation of the golden ratio, it would look like a wave wobbling around the golden ratio. This wavelength would approach the golden ratio, go past it, then come back toward it, and past it and toward it again. Each time the wave approaches the golden ratio, it gets closer and closer to that magic number.

Since you are a part of nature, you are also destined to blossom like the flowers and trees in the forest. You don't need to know the whole plan for the forest. All you need to do is keep growing as you. Your true nature will naturally blossom. This is the nature of the universe. However, as with the Fibonacci sequence, there will be wobbles, so it could feel like you're moving away from yourself and then returning home. This is also human nature. This is why you can learn to appreciate the "stuck" parts. They are part of the wave. If you "surf" the stuck parts of the wave, you will learn something from them and continue to move forward. Everything happens for a reason. Keep going, trusting in your essence, and your inner beauty will shine in everything you do.

Summary

You are by nature a spiritual being. You don't have to try to be spiritual because you already are. As spiritual beings, we are expansive light and love with infinite potential. We are here to have a human experience, which includes sadness and grief and joy and happiness. In this chapter, we explored the nature of spirit so you could better understand your true self.

1. We are individual souls emanating from One Spirit.

2. In near-death experiences, the soul can have one experience while the body has another.

3. You can strengthen your capacity for infinite trust by practicing relaxing into the giant hands of the Universe.

4. As you grow in consciousness, you will still experience life's ups and downs but with greater awareness and buoyancy.

5. Your awareness of the grand cosmic perspective can help you grow through challenges with less suffering.

6. We need both love and intention for conscious creation. The human experience is meant to be an embodiment of our soul consciousness.

7. Keep being yourself because you are destined to blossom as yourself. It is your nature.

In the next chapter, we'll discuss how to ground your spirit self in the body to feel more present and alive.

CHAPTER 8

GROUNDING THE SPIRIT

"Our awareness of Spirit changes our experience."

The moment I heard my mom's voice on the phone telling me my dad had died, I could feel myself start to dissociate—my soul floating up as words came out of my mouth, my body numb, and my vision spotty. I ran around in circles, crying and holding my head, saying, "No, no, no . . . this can't be happening. I don't know what to do. I don't know what to do!"

After some long minutes, I called myself back in. I needed to be present to access my intuition, especially my spirit's intuition. I hoped to reach out to my dad in spirit. If he was crossing over, then it was my desire to be fully aware during this precious time. I needed all my faculties to stay connected. It was hard to hear anything over the buzzing numbness in my head and body. But this was one of the most important moments, and my motivation to stay present and aware was stronger. So, I walked myself through some of the processes I described in Parts 1 and 2.

I asked myself three questions:

1. **What do you feel?**
   My answer: *I feel scared. I feel angry. I feel sad.*
   My reply to that answer: *It's okay to feel that way.*

2. **What do you feel in your body?**
   My answer: *I feel tightening in my chest, and my breath is shallow.*
   My reply to that answer: *It's okay to feel that way.*

3. Are you breathing?

My answer: *No, I'm holding my breath.*

My reply to that answer: *Keep moving your breath. Allow yourself to feel. It's okay to feel what you're feeling.*

By the time I got to the car to drive to my parents' house, I felt grounded enough to check in with Spirit. I reached out to see what was going on, and what came to me was my dad already out of his body. He was laughing in a blissful state, saying, "Oh my gosh! This is amazing!" with more rounds of laughter. He felt all peace and joy without a hint of pain or sadness. It was the most wonderful thing to witness—and here I was, upset and angry.

"Dad, what are you doing there?" I argued with him. "You need to get back in your body right now. Time is of the essence. Please get back in your body. Get back in your body. Get back in your body," I said over and over. I started pleading with God, "Please let him stay!" At the same time, I knew his body might already be beyond repair. I told my dad that if this was so, it was okay. As much as it pained me, he didn't have to return to his body in that state.

He was nowhere and everywhere. He felt like the sky, limitless, without form or embodiment. Nothing was going to stop him now.

Growing Through Grief

For the longest time, I knew that my dad and I were supposed to do something incredible together in medicine. I didn't know what this would be because he worked with the tiny particles in nanomedicine, and I was incorporating the vastness of the Spirit into my practice. Now, he had crossed over. I never imagined my great work with him would be realized while he was in Spirit.

There are life markers in our timelines that forever change us. My dad's crossing over is one of those for me. There's my life before his transition and my life after. I am different now. Life presents us all with opportunities to grow if we allow it. A friend asked me once, "How did you speak about your dad afterward without crying?" For a while, I didn't—but I spoke about him anyway through my tears because I am not afraid of being sad. Sometimes, I still cry when I talk about him, and I am still not scared of being sad. The heaviness and the infinite waves of grief remind me of the deeper love bursting through my core. We hurt because we love. We don't need to fear the depths of our love. We can use grief as a reminder of our superpower: to love and to love without fear in this moment. Whether through words, actions, gifts, or quiet prayers, we choose the love language that best communicates how we feel.

Any big life change can feel like a dying of the self—or, more accurately, a dying of the ego-self. Whether or not we choose it, we must change course. Time can feel like it's slowed down, so we have to take it step by step. This is an opportunity to be present to the juiciness of living, even when it feels terrible, and it's an opportunity to rebirth the self. When we can stay present and allow, no matter what we're experiencing, we can liberate ourselves at any moment. Major life changes can feel like the messy metamorphosis of a caterpillar becoming a butterfly.

My grandmother taught me to love myself through anything. Growing up, I occasionally heard her stories about World War II and the years after—how shrapnel flew through the bedroom window, how her baby died from dengue fever, and how burglars broke into the house. She had been through tragedy and fright, yet she never lost the sparkle in her eyes. My grandmother loved fiercely and gave generously, sharing food, crocheted items, and stories. She found joy and humor in the little things and saw the beauty in herself, which made it easy for her to see the beauty in others.

When you've been through a difficult or traumatic experience, it might sometimes feel hard to love yourself. When people ask me, "How do you start loving yourself?" I tell them about beginning with the grounding exercises I've shared in this book. I suggest choosing the ones that seem easier at first. If the mind is struggling, I recommend going to the body. My recommendation for you is the same. Do at least one exercise each day, even if it's the same one. Loving ourselves is about embracing all of ourselves no matter what we've been through. Love is that big and everlasting—that's why it's our superpower.

The Healing Power of Ceremony

Using ceremony and ritual is a beautiful and powerful way to love our way through difficult moments such as grief. I learned about this during my fellowship in Dr. Andrew Weil's integrative medicine program. Don't let the word *ceremony* intimidate you. A ceremony simply means creating sacred time and space to honor something or someone important to you. Ceremonies have a beginning to open, a middle that is the bulk of it, and an ending or a closing. One ceremony most everyone is familiar with is the birthday celebration with the birthday cake. People gather together, light candles on the cake (the opening), sing "Happy Birthday" (the middle), and cheer after the birthday honoree makes a wish and blows out the candles (the closing). It's such an elegant ceremony!

I often recommend ceremonies when people need help processing life transitions such as the death of a loved one, the birth of a child, a divorce or separation, a move, a new job—some major change or loss. A ceremony doesn't have to take long; it could be anywhere from five to twenty minutes or much longer. It's more about the intent and sincerity in the ceremony. I've seen people experience remarkable healing, lifting grief and moving stuck emotions.

The opening and closing of ceremonies are similar and involve some form of at least one of the elements of water, wind, earth, and fire. In the beginning, you are opening up sacred time and space, giving thanks and love. At the end, you close sacred time and space, again by giving thanks and love. For example, you could open by lighting a candle and saying a prayer and later close with another prayer and blowing out the candle. The middle part can be literal (such as talking with a loved one who has crossed over) or symbolic (perhaps expressing your emotions with colors in an abstract crayon drawing). Throughout the ceremony, take care to keep breathing slowly, gently, and deeply.

Table 13 on the next page provides some ideas. You can mix and match the middle parts with an opening and closing of choice.

Don't forget to give thanks and love at the end of every ceremony.

Sometimes, people ask, "Can you perform the ceremony more than once?" Yes, but not so often that it loses its significance. Instead, you can take parts of the ceremony to do more often, creating a practice rather than a ceremony—such as writing in a journal.

Table 13 – Ceremonies to Help You Grow

BEGINNING / OPENING	MIDDLE	END / CLOSING
Light a candle.	Write a letter or talk to a loved one who's crossed over.	Blow out the candle.
Say an opening prayer.	Write a letter with your intentions and burn it in a safe container (like a big pot) to send your intentions to the universe.	Sprinkle water on top of the ashes and close with a prayer.
Light incense.	Honor what you've been through by telling the story or writing it out and then shredding or burning the paper.	Blow out incense.
Light sage and let it permeate the space.	Say a poem of welcome to your new home.	Blow out the sage.
Ring a chime or a bell.	Draw a picture representing your love for someone who is ill.	Ring the chime or bell.
Play music.	Sing a song of thanksgiving.	Play music.
Spray rosewater around the space.	Use colors to draw your emotions.	Spray rosewater.
Scoop out some soil.	Plant a seed of intention.	Cover the seed with soil and water it.
Hold hands.	Jump over a small crevice to represent overcoming challenges together.	Clap and cheer.
Make a small rock pile.	Say goodbye to your old home.	Leave a flower on top of the rock pile.

The Power of Rituals

While ceremonies are performed during special times, rituals can be practiced daily to imbue more meaning into everyday life. Rituals are repeated small acts or behaviors that are part of your customary way of doing things—setting the table a certain way for meals, singing the national anthem before a sports game, a special handshake with friends, and even taco Tuesday can be a ritual.

When done with a loving intention, rituals can help us settle into whatever we are doing to be more present. Suzanne Lye, a professor of the Classics at the University of North Carolina at Chapel Hill, told me that she integrates rituals into her teaching to help her students understand their importance. "It changes the whole feeling of the class," she says. "Everyone comes in with all this stuff hanging on them from wherever they were, and my class is just one more thing they have to do. What I hope for them to do is pause and consider our classroom a special place, an expansive space that we don't allow the past or the future to encroach on. It calms everybody down. Sometimes you don't know why you feel anxious; you just feel rushed. Pausing for just ten breaths really clears things up. You literally give your brain oxygen, and it's a mental reset that's very easy to do."

Ten-Breath Reset
This simple ten-breath ritual has you pause to acknowledge the past and the future and then grounds you in the present.

- First, close your eyes.
- With your first two breaths, think about where you just were (the immediate past).
- With the third and fourth breath, think about where you will be going (the immediate future).
- On the fifth breath, be present.
- For the next five breaths, check in with yourself. Everyone can do this differently. You might focus on different aspects of your breathing. You could home in on different body parts, maybe starting with your toes and moving up to your head. You could instead notice the thoughts crossing your mind and observe your state of mind at this moment. Again, everyone will have their way of checking in—it's up to you.
- On the tenth breath, open your eyes.

You can practice this simple ritual alone or with others, whether at the beginning of a class, event, meal, or as a way to start and end the day. You will find that your rituals infuse more meaning into your everyday life and find it easier to see the signs in your daily life as you go about your business.

Coincidences or Signs?

My friend Maudy Fowler is a spiritual consultant. She told me and my family that my dad would leave feathers on our paths to let us know he was thinking of us. Soon enough, my cousin Christina found a feather on a nature trail. She smiled and thought of my dad—but then, the skeptical part of her mind took hold, and Christina remembers thinking, *Oh, but it's so small! Is it really a sign?* Literally three steps later, she saw a bigger feather and heard my dad laughing.

The same thing happened to my sister. She saw little feathers on the ground, which made her smile. But it was also springtime, and she thought, *They're so little. It's probably a coincidence.* Then she asked our dad, "Please leave me big signs that I can't miss because I could really use them." Over the next week, she found three ginormous feathers—one near her home was the biggest she'd ever seen, measuring sixteen inches.

My youngest sister also sent out a sincere plea for a sign. She was on the other side of the world when our dad passed and felt an extra layer of grief being so far away. That same day, she had seen multiple butterflies and thought of my dad, but she was uncertain. As one of the butterflies was flying away, she thought, *Dad, if you can hear me, then get that butterfly to land on me, and I'll know.* The butterfly was about one hundred feet away when it turned around, flew back, and landed on her. She says tears streamed down her face in grief, gratitude, and awe.

What's the difference between a coincidence and a miracle? They're the same thing really, but one has more meaning because of your awareness and perspective. Again, we all crave meaning. There are signs everywhere helping us—it's simply a matter of learning how to see them. The more signs and miracles we recognize, the more frequently they occur. Our awareness changes our experience. The following exercise can help you shift your awareness by trusting your heart.

Exercise: Reading Your Heart

This exercise expands on the Hand on Heart exercise from Ways to Access Your Body's Wisdom on page 70.

1. Place one hand or both on your heart and bring your awareness to your heart field. (The palms of our hands take in a lot of sensory input, so your attention will naturally follow their placement.)

2. Next, you'll need a comparison to calibrate how you read your heart. Note that once you're used to reading your heart, you don't have to repeat this step each time. Pick a joyful moment or a happy place in your life. Practice feeling into your body, especially your heart field. Note what joy feels like in your heart field (an opening, expansion, relaxation, or brightening). Then, pick a somewhat sad or frustrating moment. For the purposes of this calibration exercise, don't pick the most intense moment. Notice what the mildly sad or frustrating emotion feels like in your heart field (a closing or shielding, contraction, tensing, or dulling). Once you've felt the difference between the two states, you'll have a good gauge for what the opening and closing of your heart field feels like. To reset before going on to the next step, embrace all emotions, hug yourself in, take a deep sigh breath, and shake your body out.

3. Now, you can ask your heart anything. Do you have any worries or questions about a particular situation? Your heart will help you look from its higher perspective of love and provide direction. See your situation from various perspectives. Whatever rings true for your heart will create a heart opening. You can also scan different parts of your life, such as work, family, rest, play, and nourishment. An area that needs tending will create a heart opening. Your heart can tell you where the healing is, and it will lead you with love for yourself and others.

As you practice this, be mindful: Are you listening to your heart or a craving from the mind or body? I've taught this exercise to kids, teens, and adults. A shy child learned to be more decisive, teens were able to make more heart-informed choices when it came to making friends, and adults were able to worry less as they learned to trust themselves.

Fearless Living

One of the messages I received from my dad in spirit was: "Enjoy all of your days because the end is not the end." The feelings I get from my dad in pure spirit form are infinite bliss and love. Any grief or hurt he carried in his heart has dissipated. He feels peaceful, while the rest of us here still feel all kinds of emotions. The strange thing, though, is that sometimes I miss the ups and downs with my dad. Being able to feel in multisensory ways is magnificent. Life is like a great multidimensional movie we are living. Afterward, we will marvel at it and say, "What a movie!" So, enjoy your days, enjoy your movie, and see if you can steer it toward more love for yourself, others, and the planet.

Since my dad died, I no longer fear death in the same way. Now, it's more a fear of not living. I hope to live in the moment no matter how hard it is. I urge you, too, to not be afraid to share who you are with the world because you are a part of the fabric of the universe. Don't be afraid to bring who you are into your life and get the most out of every moment. Ask yourself:

- How would I like to live in this moment despite the difficulties I'm facing?
- How can I make the best of it right now?
- How can I bring my unique gifts and personality to this moment?

I'm also not afraid to enjoy life and pursue my passions in a bigger way. Why not? When you go through a big loss and then realize there is no loss in Spirit, it moves you to bring all of yourself into living. No more holding back. It's time to bare your soul.

What Is Forgiveness?

Let's clear up some of the misunderstandings about forgiveness. First, it is for you; forgiveness sets you free. You know you've been able to forgive when thinking about the person or situation no longer has a grip on you. It no longer makes you cringe and feel bad. You can remember the story, but it has lost its intensity. You've released its power over you. You can now move forward. But if you still have a cringe or visceral reaction to the person or situation, you haven't fully processed it and let it go. Forgiveness helps us free ourselves from believing the past can hold us back.

Second, true forgiveness encourages you to accept your authentic experience. You can't bypass what you've been through. To ensure you are honoring and tending to yourself, start in the present. You may have feelings such as anger, sadness, or grief. Be a loving, nonjudgmental witness to your feelings—as we discussed in chapter 5. Complete acceptance of yourself as you are now is part of the process of true forgiveness. You don't have to express each of your emotions in the world (although doing so might be helpful); acknowledging what you feel and expressing this to yourself is enough. Seeing and hearing yourself is vital to self-healing. Get help with this part if you need it. With true forgiveness, we honor our emotions and see and hear ourselves as we are in this moment, including unprocessed past emotions.

Third, forgiveness is not about forgetting. "Forgive and forget" may not serve you. Forgiveness is about love and your desire to care for yourself and live sustainably. That may mean making changes in your life to love yourself better. Forgiveness helps us learn from the past and move forward consciously.

One of my favorite definitions of forgiveness is from *A Course in Miracles*, the book psychologist Helen Schucman scribed in a process of divine inner dictation. *A Course in Miracles* says, "Forgiveness is the healing of the perception of separation."[1] In other words, true forgiveness is forgiving yourself for believing that you or anyone else is separate from the Oneness. True forgiveness is remembering who you are, remembering your true self as a divine being, an emanation of the Oneness. Clearly understood, regardless of whether you forgive yourself or another—and vice versa—all are part of the Oneness. The light of Oneness is eternal, so whatever terrible thing anyone experiences, that light can never be put out. We are all part of that Oneness. *A Course in Miracles* also teaches that "Everything is love ... or a call for love." This means that everything is either *an expression of* love or *a call for* love. It's all about love.

Let's unpack True Forgiveness in a Three-Step Process.

Step 1: Wake up to the knowing that you are the creator of your life. What you feel will be mirrored in your outer world—as within, so without. This may not be easy at first, so it's important to let yourself feel however you feel. Life consists of mysteries we can't understand as humans. Some people are born into privilege, while others are dealt a difficult hand. Human-made cultural creations such as racism, sexism, and prejudice can be the cause of injustices—but regardless of what you've been born into, you can choose to wake up and become a co-creator of your life. Being a co-creator means you create with the Oneness. We start from within. So, if we hope to see peace in the world, we need to feel peace in ourselves first. If we hope to see love in the world, we need to love. Love and peace must be in us before we can see it outside in the world.

Step 2: Be willing to see another perspective, a grander perspective. We can remember to see ourselves as part of the divine whole of life, not separate from it. To wake up to true forgiveness, open your mind to the Oneness you've always been a part of and will forever be. When we suffer, it's because we've forgotten this connection. We are each a unique and essential thread in the entire tapestry of all life.

The ego often resists this truth. It's a protection mechanism because the unknown tends to trigger fear in the ego. Your ego will try to protect you from further pain by reminding you of your hurt and keeping you in the limited box of what it knows. However, the pain of forgetting your true self is far greater. When you remember who you are, you're no longer lost at sea. You realize you're in the middle of the vast ocean of Oneness. When you know who you are, you are willing to accept and process human hurts. In truth, you hurt because you love—you love yourself and others, but you have forgotten that you *are* love. When you remember your divine nature, you may still experience physical, mental, and emotional hurt, but you won't suffer in the same way. It's easier when you know you are Love.

Step 3: Ask for divine help to remember your true nature. We cannot do this with the ego alone. Asking the Oneness to help you forgive is one of the best prayers. Allow yourself the gift of receiving help with forgiveness. The human mind does not understand how to forgive completely, so we pray to remember that we are all part of the Oneness. When we do, so much healing can occur in body, mind, and spirit. Physical pain can lift, mental and emotional pain can lift, discomfort lifts—and we are at peace.

Keep in mind that if the pain does not immediately lift, it's not a judgment on you but part of the forgiveness process, of letting yourself be. You are free to be you, however you are, without any judgment. You free yourself when you are no longer weighed down by your perception of yourself as a victim. You realize your infinite potential through spirit, and in that is the joy, peace, and love that is healing. In short, the process of true forgiveness is as follows:

- Wake up to the knowing that you co-create your life with the Oneness.
- Be willing to see a grander perspective.
- Ask for divine help.

Addressing Guilt

I used to feel guilty a lot, not for any particular reason. It was more not feeling good enough—like I didn't try my best, or I should have done more or something differently. I felt guilty for being me. This had me looking for ways to shake the guilty feeling. Now, I realize feeling guilty is a red flag for being out of balance and a reminder to forgive. Guilt goes hand in hand with fear. When we feel guilty, we tend to look elsewhere for the guilt in others or to contain it and not feel it by numbing out or overcontrolling. Remember that overhelping or people-pleasing can be a way of controlling. All the while, the remedy is within—the light of the soul. There, we remember ourselves as part of all creation. and there, we can ask Spirit to guide us. Releasing our guilt and our projection of it onto others are also part of forgiveness.

A Forgiveness Ritual

You can incorporate forgiveness into your daily practice with the following prayer, and you can use any of its lines as a mantra during sitting meditation, a mindful walk, yoga practice, or another quiet time for reflection. Keep a sincere and open mind as you say these words. I recommend spending about fifteen minutes twice a day with this, but whatever timeframe you can give is worthwhile, even a few minutes.

Dear Universe,

Let me perceive true forgiveness.

Help me to

See through the eyes of Love

Hear through the ears of Love

Feel through the heart of Love

Speak through the voice of Love

Understand through the mind Love

And align my will with Love.

Help me forgive so that I can remember the Truth

that I am always part of the Oneness.

Please help me to remember who I am when I have forgotten.

I am One with the Divinity.

I am loved and

I am Love.

Thank you.

You could also try reflecting on someone while you say this prayer or see what comes up when you reflect on the prayer's first line, "Let me perceive true forgiveness." See what guilt comes up, yours or the projection of another's. See what fears or hurts come up. You might become aware of that tug between the mind and soul. Let them all be; let each breath and each repetition of the mantra steer you toward the light that you are. As you continue to practice, you may feel a lightening in your body and the relief of a burden being lifted. Forgiveness liberates us and reminds us of the essence of being human.

Ubuntu, the Essence of Being Human

I'd like to share the transcript of a moving talk I came across on video from Archbishop Desmond Tutu explaining the philosophy of Ubuntu:[2]

Let me tell you we have something in our African community, something that is difficult to put into English. It's called Ubuntu. Ubuntu is the essence of being human, and it says, a solitary human being is a contradiction in terms. I can't be a human being on my lonesome. I wouldn't know how to speak as a human being, I wouldn't know how to think as a human being, I wouldn't know how to walk as a human being. I have to learn from other human beings how to be human.

And so, Ubuntu says my humanity is bound to yours. I am only because you are. And we will then see a person is a person through other persons. And that we need this communal harmony if we're going to survive at all. And anger and revenge and bitterness are corrosive of this harmony.

And you know it. You experience it when you are angry at somebody. It does something to your tum-tum. And you, it does something to your blood pressure.

So, forgiving is not actually being altruistic. You're not being nice to the other guy when you forgive. You're actually being nice to yourself."

I was talking to a friend once about a situation with loved ones that involved misunderstandings and hurts on all sides. We had different opinions, and all felt judged by one another. My friend asked me, "What would it take for you to heal from this?" I paused and let the question sink in. "Do nothing," I answered, "and accept their hurts and my hurts, too, because we are no more and no less worthy of love regardless of what we feel or have been through. Everything is love or a call for love." Literally, the moment I said that I received an intuitive message, and the issue I was concerned about dissolved. Once I could see and again feel that we are all part of the Oneness, the problem dissipated—a small miracle. Stepping back to get a grander perspective, I saw there was never really a problem in the first place. Love is our true nature. The soul knows this truth. It's a matter of remembering this over and over again.

Summary

Our awareness of Spirit changes our experience. Grounding the Spirit's expansiveness into our human being requires love and compassion.

1. You can grow through grief, which can feel like a dying of the self (ego). You have to let go and step into the next moment continuously. As you do, your grief can become a joyful, loving grief.

2. A ceremony creates sacred time and space to honor something or someone important to you. Ceremonies have an opening, a middle, and a closing. For example, lighting a candle, singing happy birthday, and then blowing out the candle is a simple ceremony.

3. Rituals are daily practices you find meaningful. They help you settle into whatever you are doing so that you are more present. Setting the table for dinner and praying before meals is an example of a daily ritual.

4. The more you notice signs and miracles, the more often they occur. Your awareness changes your experience.

5. Don't be afraid of living, even during the challenging times. Ask yourself, *How can I make the best of it right now? How can I bring my unique gifts to this moment?*

6. Forgiveness is for giving yourself freedom; it sets you free.

7. Forgiveness includes forgiving yourself for misperceiving yourself as separate from the Oneness. Forgiveness is remembering your divine nature and the divine nature of all beings. You can ask the Divine for help with forgiveness.

8. Ubuntu is an African philosophy and way of life that says my humanity is bound with yours. It is the essence of being human. Ubuntu also sees forgiveness as being kind to yourself. Humans survive only in harmony.

Now that you understand how to feel more present with Spirit, we can turn to Spirit for intuitive guidance. Spirit is our compass.

CHAPTER 9

YOUR SPIRIT AS YOUR COMPASS

*"That still small voice inside of you that's always
loving and encouraging is Spirit's guidance."*

Receiving messages directly from Spirit made me nervous at first.
When patients came to me for consults and osteopathic treatments, I felt guided, as if an angelic presence showed me exactly what
to do. We never talked about *that* in medical school! I kept quiet about
it for a couple of reasons: How could I be sure if it was real? And what
would people think of me?

Listening to Spirit takes trust in ourselves and the Universe. A part of
the mind may not be sure it's receiving actual guidance—the "am I crazy?"
part. But the soul experiences this guidance as a resonance and a knowing.
Sometimes, we choose to listen to Spirit; other times, we don't. We all have
free will. I encourage you to conduct mini experiments, taking note of
whether life flows better when you listen to Spirit versus when you don't.

As for what people might think of you taking guidance from Spirit,
that's something for us to see clearly and grow beyond. One day, an
energy healer helped me with this. I told her I felt lonely being different.
She told me my loneliness wasn't something she could treat because it
was part of my life path, "to learn to be alone but not lonely." That statement changed my life. I never felt lonely again because I understood
there was a deeper purpose at work and decided to embrace Spirit's
guidance fully. This is true for everyone. You can also turn to Spirit's
guidance to help set you on your true path.

Your "Extra Senses"

Messages from Spirit are everywhere. If you're an empath or a highly sensitive person, recognizing those messages can be challenging because all kinds of stimuli get your attention and can easily overwhelm you. The good news is that you can learn to sort and decipher the data coming through your senses. If you'd like, review the "quiz" in chapter 3 to determine what kinds of intuition you currently have an inclination for. Here, we're going to expand on that and discuss ways to develop your intuitive senses further. Here's an overview of what I call your "extra-sensory system" to help you with this.

Sight. What catches your eye? Whatever it is, there's a reason for it. I learned a great exercise from Dr. Jacob Liberman, an optometrist and vision and light researcher.[1] Spend at least 15 minutes, and up to several hours if you like, following the light of your eye, and as you notice things, consider what you notice as your responsibility for that moment and meet it with love.

I did this once on a walk in the woods. I found medicinal herbs and mushrooms along the way and bits of litter mixed in with the fallen leaves. I tucked the litter into a bag I had and dropped it into the appropriate bins later. This is a simple example of what can happen when we meet what we see with love.

Signs that have meaning for you may catch your eye. Feathers, birds, and butterflies are often recognized as whispers from Spirit. You may see words pop up somewhere that are meant to guide you. For example, you could flip through this book and see what page and words catch your eye. Colors you're drawn to are also significant; they tend to represent strengths we possess. We can get a sense of what colors are in someone's energy field (aura) from the colors that look good on them. Colors we find repelling represent qualities or life areas that need rebalancing. When we're flowing with life, we feel comfortable with any color. Note also how life can feel devoid of color when it is off balance, like a season of gray days.

Here's a table of colors and the qualities generally associated with them, and for some, also the corresponding chakra (or energy center):

Table 14 - Understanding the Meanings of Colors

COLOR	MEANING	CHAKRA
Red	Grounding, will, vitality	Root
Orange	Abundance, play, joy	Sacral
Yellow	Light, confident, sunny	Solar plexus
Lime	Cleansing, grace, rebirth	
Green	Love, compassion, wholeness	Heart
Turquoise	Immunity, water, freedom	
Blue	Breathe, trust, peace	Throat
Indigo	Inspiration, imagination, vision	Third eye
Violet	Spirit, serenity, guidance	Crown
Purple	Grace, gentleness, sleep	
Magenta	Birth, gratitude, dawn	
Carmine	Beauty, reconnection	

Body Sensations. Sometimes, the sensations you feel in your body will be clues from Spirit. Maybe someone tells you something, and the truth you hear gives you goosebumps or chills. These goosebumps are different from the ones you get when you're scared or nervous because you also feel a heart-opening and lightness and expansion in your body—and that's confirmation from the Universe.

Here are some other body sensations you might feel when Spirit sends you a message of confirmation. Remember that you'll also experience an expansion in your heart, body, and energy field:

- Goosebumps or a chill in your spine
- A wave of perspiration or warmth, like a warm blanket of air
- The wind at your neck or hair
- Butterflies in your belly
- The heart racing
- The heart opening

- A sense of urgency

- A nudge to do something

These various body sensations won't be ongoing if they're a message from Spirit. Instead, they'll be transient, like a wave passing through you. The next time you get one of these momentary sensations, pause to check in with yourself. Is there an expansion in your heart, body, or energy field? Reflect on what just happened. Did someone say something important? What were you looking at? What thought went through your mind? Is there a coincidence in what just occurred?

Smell. Like your eyes, your olfactory nerve is an extension of your brain. Smells trigger the olfactory nerve and send messages directly to the limbic system, the area of the brain that processes emotions and memory. Smell is an efficient way to communicate a message because it brings up specific associations and memories. A single scent can trigger so many subconscious connections before your conscious mind can make sense of it. Many people didn't realize how important their sense of smell is until they had it taken away with COVID-19.

If you smell something and you're not sure where it came from, pay attention. Once, my siblings smelled our dad's cooking months after he passed. They weren't making the foods they smelled, which made them smile and think, *Hi, Dad! Is that you? Thanks for saying hello!*

I know a bodyworker who often smells things when she's working on the energy center associated with the person's liver and gallbladder, organs that are important in digestion and detoxification. She can smell when a person's body is saturated with a particular drug or herb or with coffee or chocolate. The ability to smell emotions is called a "synesthetic response." A physician colleague of mine can smell when someone is stressed, rushed, afraid, or in an open-hearted state.

Sound. As I mentioned in chapter 3, hearing a buzzing sound can be a message from Spirit. This is different from chronic tinnitus or the ringing in your ears from a physical injury, virus, or another physical problem. This is a buzzing that comes and goes, like goosebumps. It's as if your ears are picking up on a distant radio station. Sometimes, the sound lasts a couple of days but isn't loud enough to be entirely distracting. When I hear a faint ringing or buzzing, I know there's an important message coming through from Spirit, and to hear it, I've got to get quiet.

If you hear a ringing or buzzing, tune into the frequency, like you're adjusting the dial on an old radio. Ask the Universe, "Is there a message I'm supposed to receive?" Then, get very still and listen to the whisper behind your thoughts. You can think of your thoughts being broadcast on loudspeakers while the guidance from Spirit comes through as the whispers behind your thoughts. That's why it's important to get quiet, so you can hear these whispers. The still, small voice inside you is always loving and encouraging. Spirit hopes for us to flow with life and gently guides us this way. It usually won't be louder than our surface thoughts, so we have to get quiet and choose to listen.

I notice the whispers when I'm overwhelmed by intense emotions. Sometimes they say, *It's okay. Everything is going to be okay.* Other times, they say, *This feels like a big deal, but it's not as big a deal as it seems. Let this go. There are more important things in your life to tend to.*

You can practice turning down the volume of your dominant thoughts to hear the whispers by imagining you're turning down the volume knob on your thoughts. Then, let your butterfly thoughts flit freely without the pressure of judgment. Imagine tiny little butterflies coming and going as well—so small you might have missed them. These tiny butterflies represent the whispers behind your thoughts. Imagine another volume knob that can turn up the sound on these whispers. Be quiet, patient, and still so you can hear.

Knowing. Sometimes, Spirit's guidance comes as a knowing. This is when you get a feeling inside and can't explain how you know something—you just *know.* This knowing is different from having to be right, because your inner knowing doesn't need validation. It's also not about your ego thinking you're smarter than others. It's when your heart, mind, and spirit are aligned in a neutral and certain knowing.

I see many parents who have this knowing when it comes to their kids. They know when their kids aren't feeling well or acting themselves. I find the more parents calmly and confidently follow this knowing, the easier things are for them. You may have this knowing in one area of your life but not others. The great news is that if you're intuitive in one area, you already know how to tap into it. As you allow that receptivity into the rest of your life, you'll feel more balanced, and life will get easier.

Also, take note that your extra senses can work together. For example, you could smell something and have an inner knowing at the same time or get goosebumps and hear the whispered message at the same time. As I already mentioned, one of your extra senses could be stronger than the others; it also happens that the strength of your extra senses could vary by situation.

Four Common Types of Meditation

A surefire way to develop your intuition is through the practice of meditation. Let's look at four common types of meditation. You can practice one type alone or blend them.

1. **Breathing meditation.** The word *inspire* comes from the Latin *inspirare,* meaning "to breathe or blow into," and came into use in the 14th century when it meant "to breathe in spirit," a meaning it still carries. When we place a soft focus on our breath, we align our mind, body, and spirit, while the awareness of our breath helps us embrace ourselves in the moment. As you focus on your breath in breathing meditation, intentionally breathe in love and breathe out what no longer serves you. (See chapter 2 for other breathing exercises.)

2. **Visualization.** How would you like to feel? What is your heart's desire? With visualization, you play the scenario out like a movie in your imagination while consciously breathing along. Really feel the experience, too, with full-bodied emotion in your whole being. Once you've fully imagined your heart's desire, let it go. Now, trust what unfolds.

3. **Prayer, or talking meditation.** I consider prayer a talking meditation. We ask for help from the Universe and give thanks for the help we know will be given. We are never alone in this universe, so ask for help whenever you need it—and be willing to receive it.

4. Listening meditation. It's hard to listen to Spirit when there's so much chatter in our heads. But you can use your breath to shift your awareness to the quiet and calm center inside you where the whisper of guidance will always be loving and supportive.

Getting quiet and listening to Spirit is so rewarding. I set aside time to listen each morning and night. When I first started meditating in my twenties, it was tricky because of the distracting tension in my body and looping thoughts in my mind. Meditation tested my patience. But I learned that grounding the body, mind, and spirit at the start makes a difference, as does centering in the heart. Staying committed to the practice also makes it easier.

Meditation has helped me write this book. I paused to listen for Spirit's guidance whenever I felt unsure or stuck. The practice I used was simple and might be helpful to you, too.

- First, get quiet—really quiet—somewhere away from the usual distractions. Sit comfortably, whether cross-legged or with your feet flat on the floor; use a pillow for comfort if needed. Ideally, keep your spine aligned. Getting quiet and turning the volume of your thoughts down can be difficult at first, especially if you're not used to it—which leads to the next step.

- Remind yourself that you are more than your mind and your body. You are a soul. When we meditate, we prioritize the soul and allow it to receive answers from Spirit.

- Listen. With all your "extra" senses, listen and be patient in the silence. Spirit's communication may come in the form of words or as a knowing, a feeling, or a vision. Be open to receiving what comes. Spirit's answers will always be encouraging, supportive, and loving. If the information isn't encouraging, your ego thoughts are still too loud. Stay quiet, patient, and receptive.

Spirit often gives me the message to "do nothing," which doesn't mean lying on the couch waiting for life to happen—although if you need rest, that is what "do nothing" means. When Spirit answers me with guidance to do nothing, it usually means don't resist the experience

I'm having and trust Spirit's support. Remember the "be-do-have" concept from Part 2? Doing nothing requires that same prioritization of *being*. To do nothing in this sense is about allowing life to be as it is. Instead of holding tight to our notions about how life should be, we allow it to show us. When we can let life *be* in this way, we are freed. To reiterate, doing nothing is *not* passive. Instead, it is a relaxed strength, which is stronger than a tense strength.[2] In doing nothing we are listening to and placing our trust in the Stillness, where the potency of Spirit resides. From that Stillness, anything is possible, so by doing nothing (*be*ing in Stillness) we can create (*do*ing with purpose) with ease (flowing with abundance).

Your Life's Guidance

Life itself guides us in incredible ways. In Part 1, we looked at physical symptoms as your body's way of communicating; similarly, your life also communicates with you. This may not be easy to see at first, but once you realize it, you start to see the beauty in every moment, even the hard ones. The hard moments trigger uncomfortable emotional reactions that also show us where the healing is. In other words, your triggers are showing you where the healing is.

When something doesn't seem to go your way, maybe it's not meant to. Everything happens for a reason, and everything is for our soul growth. You may not immediately know what those reasons are and what growth you'll experience, but understanding that there is a bigger picture is helpful. Realize that the hard times are stepping stones to something better, and expect amazing things no matter what. Challenges also add interest to your story. When my oldest was in elementary school reading the books in *A Series of Unfortunate Events,* I asked her if she liked them since something bad always happened. She looked at me and said, "Mommy, it wouldn't be a good story if nothing bad happened."

After my dad died—one of the hardest moments in my life—I decided to spend the rest of my life loving as much as I could. That includes loving myself. I hope to get the most out of every moment, whether sitting quietly alone, making dinner, or talking to a patient. Each moment is precious. Once I started looking at life through this lens, things shifted rapidly. My husband and I bonded on an even deeper level, projects that were dragging gained momentum, and I feel more confident out in the world.

My Rule of Three

To help myself flow with life, I came up with what I call "my rule of three," which goes like this: If I attempt to do something three times but am somehow blocked each time, I pause and ask myself, *How can I look at this differently?* It might be that I need to relax before going forward or that I need to consider a different path altogether. Pausing and reassessing like this helps us listen to life's guidance—this way, life doesn't have to throw a tantrum to get our attention.

Once, I was trying to call in an order for specific remedies. I tried to make the phone call three times, and each time, I couldn't connect: first, there was static on the line; the second time, I had to answer another call; and the third time, I accidentally called the wrong number. I decided to call a colleague instead to consult about the remedies I was looking for, and she told me about a different company with better-quality remedies. That outcome confirmed that I was listening to my life's guidance when I paused calling after the third attempt.

Healing with Grace

Grace is love without judgment. Grace is often discussed in a religious context, but it isn't limited to religion. It belongs to Spirit, and we are all spiritual beings. Grace disrupts logic. It operates in the quantum, opening up nonlinear pathways and gateways to miracles. With grace, you move forward because there is no judgment to hold you back. Grace and forgiveness go hand in hand, allowing you to step into the possibilities in each new moment. To love without judgment is to tap into an infinite love.

The next time you're frustrated, consider giving yourself some grace. I've seen that we need to give ourselves grace especially when we're starting something new in life—a new job, a new move, a new family. Doing something new can feel awkward or raise anxiety at first. My patient Amy felt this way when she was about to make a big move after a difficult divorce. She was in a rush to get settled and fell back into her old habit of beating herself up for not having it all finished already. I reminded her to give herself some grace. When she heard the word *grace*, she lit up. "That's right!" she said, "Give myself some grace." With that shift, she exhaled and relaxed into life's timing.

Healing with Hope

Hope is a powerful force for good. More than a wish, hope is trusting that everything will work out in alignment with the Universe. Hope helps us keep going. But we have to choose hope. Bumps in the road are inevitable, whether minor annoyances or huge roadblocks. We all meet these, but we can easily fall into despair without hope.

Once, my cousin was in a coma after a terrible car accident. The doctors said it was not likely he would regain normal functioning. My dad, also a physician, spoke with all the specialists to help explain the circumstances to my aunt and uncle. I remember the conversation my dad had with me before talking to them. "It doesn't look good," he told me. "What do you think I should say?" I was a new pediatrician and a new mom at the time. It wasn't like my dad to ask for my medical opinion then. But this was different. It was a medical situation and a family situation. I felt the weight of his responsibility. I understood that his words would impact how we all would hold the moment and the future that would unfold. "Whatever you say, do not lose hope," I told my dad. There was a possibility of things turning around—a slim one, yet it existed. If we take away hope, what else is there? My aunt's hope and strength were unwavering. It was a long and difficult road. Months later, against the odds, my cousin opened his eyes. He had to learn how to walk, talk, and eat again, but he did it. The doctors and medical staff called it a miracle.

I love this description of hope from Neale Donald Walsch in his book *Home with God*: "Hope is a statement of your highest desire. It is the announcement of your grandest dream. Hope is thought made divine." Whenever I read that passage, I'm inspired never to give up.

What does hope feel like in your body? For me, it feels like beams of sunshine emanating from my heart and throughout my being. The feeling of hope releases the tension that grips us when we worry. Cultivate this trusting-knowing feeling of hope moment by moment. Let your body beam with hope, and you will get through anything.

Communicating with Loved Ones Who Have Crossed Over

My grandmother was a true matriarch, the glue that held our extended family together. I loved hanging out with her. Although she crossed over years ago and is no longer in physical form, I still talk to her almost every day. I still feel connected to her. I encourage everyone who's had a loved one pass away to be open to communicating with them still. Know that when you're thinking of your loved one, they're thinking of you, too. The connection is automatic. It's a matter of opening up to this and becoming aware of the relationship you still have.

Hope and trust will help you open your awareness to the messages from loved ones who have passed away. I've seen people hope for such signs but then miss them, though the signs are there. This is when developing trust makes a huge difference. You trust that *you can* receive messages and that *you will,* in divine timing.

Communication with those who've crossed over goes both ways. If there are things you would like to say that were unsaid while the person was living, go ahead and tell them now. They will hear you. Trust this. It will help soothe and heal your grief, too.

I had a patient named Leslie who was depressed. She'd lost interest in doing things and going anywhere, although she used to love traveling. Her friends convinced her to travel one state over to visit them. They also lived near me and encouraged her to see me. When we met, I learned that her father had passed away years ago. She said she didn't miss him. They had not been on good terms, so their relationship had many loose ends. Leslie was still angry at her father for things he'd said and done and for the things he didn't say and didn't do. I gave her an assignment: to write a letter to her father expressing everything she hadn't said. She was reluctant, but she did this. A few weeks later, her friend Mary told me Leslie was vacationing in Europe. Her depression had lifted. You never know what will happen when you address what's most important in your heart.

Since my dad crossed over, my niece has been able to communicate with him easily. She says, "It's like he has a door to my heart and can pop in and out to say, 'I love you!'" You can do this, too. Here are a few simple steps to get you started:

1. Center yourself in your heart field (in Part 1), and breathe into it.

2. Staying aware of your heart center, say this mantra: "I hope to hear from *(name of your loved one)*. I trust I can hear from *(name of your loved one)*. I trust in divine timing."

3. Let go of the outcome. Be patient and trust.

4. Be open to how Spirit will deliver its messages to you.

Guidance from Your Dreamworld

In our dreams, we are uninhibited by space, time, and the body, and we can also access universal knowledge. Many people have been inspired and guided by their dreams. Einstein came up with the theory of relativity, Larry Page found the algorithm for Google, and Mary Shelley dreamed the tale of Frankenstein. Because the rational mind doesn't understand how the dreamworld works, it may fight against it. That's understandable, but to move forward, we must accept that life is full of great mysteries. How egotistical to think we humans could have it all figured out. It's wise instead to get comfortable with the fact that life is mysterious. This is part of its beauty. One of life's mysteries is our dreamworld.

Here are a few guidelines to help you begin tapping into your dream life[3]:

- Start with the intention that you'd like to work with your dreams.

- Have a pen and some paper on your nightstand.

- When you first wake in the morning, write down anything you can recall from your dreams. Also, write down the strongest emotions you associate with a dream and any images or symbols you saw that strongly impacted you.

- If you can't remember any dreams when you wake, write instead in a stream-of-consciousness flow for ten minutes. Write down whatever comes up, no matter how weird.

Here are a few suggestions to help you interpret your dreams. Remember that dreams are often symbolic and sometimes literal. Also, keep in mind that your dream is your dream, which means there are no hard rules for dream interpretation. I can only suggest ways to approach your dreamworld.

- Consider what the images in your dream mean to you. For example, if a cat was in your dream, what does a cat mean in your waking life? If you had a cat that made you feel safe and loved while growing up, perhaps this is what the cat in the dream represents for you.

- Give the dream a title. If your dream were a chapter in a book, what would you title it?

- Think about what is going on in your life right now and how elements in your dream correspond to what is happening. Are there discomforts you can let go of? Somewhere you could use more courage? Our dreams can shed more light and provide more clarity about any area of our lives. You may be surprised by what comes up.

- Meditating on your dream can help you access deeper meanings. There can be layers of interpretation to a dream, starting with the obvious and often literal surface meaning. There is also the symbolic meaning. A listening meditation helps with dream interpretation. Set the intention, *If I need to receive any information, I am open to receiving it*, and wait in silence for whatever emerges. It may be a thought, a feeling, or another kind of knowing. Whatever comes up, write it down because the details may be fleeting.

Occasionally, your dream may be a message for someone else. To help determine this, consider the "main character" in your dream. Is the spotlight on you or someone else? If you think your dream is a message for another person, ask and meditate on the question. Spirit works in mysterious ways and might call on you to help another in this way. Sometimes, the person needs to be told, but other times, simply sending them loving thoughts is all that needs to be done.

I've dreamt about people I haven't seen in decades and wouldn't even know how to contact anymore. Usually, I find all that is needed from me is to say a prayer for them. When I get a clear call to say something to the person I've dreamt about, it feels like an inner itch or a nagging feeling that won't go away. It's something I have to do. I know this is so when my mind and body are aligned with the feeling of necessity.

I've also had premonitions. A few months before my dad passed, for example, I had a dream that something was happening to him, but it wasn't clear what. I struggled with the dream for many months. When my dad died, I felt I could have prevented his death but failed. I didn't share this with many people because it was too hard to explain then. During the funeral service, when I stood by my dad's coffin looking down at his frozen body, I had this knowing-feeling that all was meant to be and that there was nothing I was supposed to have done differently. The dream I'd had was information for me—a heads up, so to speak. I wasn't meant to change the course of events. That realization was a bittersweet moment, with a wave of peace and joy washing over the canyon of sadness.

You will be the best interpreter of your dreams. If you need some guidance, you can turn to one of the many resources on dreams, dream archetypes, and dream interpretation that are out there. I've included some of my favorites in the resources section at the back of this book. You could also consult a spiritual consultant to help you with your dreams.

Summary

Spirit is always here for you, waiting for you to notice its messages. That still small voice inside of you that's always loving and encouraging is Spirit's guidance. The best way to attune yourself to its guidance is in stillness.

1. Listen to the still, small voice inside you, the loving whispers behind your louder thoughts.

2. Sometimes, doing nothing but accepting life as it is and trusting life is all that is needed. *Do nothing and all is done* is infinite trust.

3. Whatever triggers you is also showing you where the healing is.

4. Everything that happens in your life is for your soul's growth. When something doesn't go your way, pause and reassess with this in mind.

5. Spend the rest of your life loving as much as you can.

6. Grace is love without judgment, and it moves you forward because there are no judgments to hold you back. Grace disrupts logic and opens quantum gateways.

7. Hope connects your thoughts with your heart and Spirit.

8. Loved ones who have crossed over haven't left you. Hope and trust can help you stay connected with them.

9. Your dreamworld is a rich source of spiritual connection and intuition.

Now, let's put everything we've looked at in this book together and celebrate the intuition of your body, mind, and spirit—your multidimensional nature.

Exercises for the Intuitive Spirit

Send a Rainbow

I love this practice, which was inspired by a deck of yoga cards I used with my kids. Once, when my oldest was five and I was leaving her room before bedtime after playing with the deck together, she pleaded with me to pick one more card. I pulled the rainbow card and told her, "I'm sending you a rainbow!" I placed my palms up and imagined a rainbow of energy from me to her. She said, "Oh, Mommy! I can feel it!" I was surprised. I wasn't used to other people feeling things the way I do. Since then, I've discovered that many people, kids and adults, can feel these energetic rainbows.

Here's how you can send a rainbow to someone:

- Shake out your body to help ground and center yourself.
- Rub your palms together to wake up the energy points there.
- Extend your palms outward and imagine a rainbow spreading from your palms to the other person, whether they're in the same room or far away.
- Alternatively, you could imagine the rainbow spanning out from your heart center to the other person's heart center.

We are meant to spread blessings wherever we are. You could send a rainbow not only to people but also to animals, plants, a home, a community. When we give love, we never run out. The earth needs our blessings.

Add Color to Your Life

In a TED Talk by designer Ingrid Fetell Lee called "Where Joy Hides and How to Find It," Lee shares abundant of research that shows the impact colors have on us: a colorful world brings us joy. The white, bare walls and neutral-colored furnishings of most office buildings, hospitals, and schools give us no joy, but nature's colors soothe. When we bring more color into our lives, we create lives with more joy. Here are some ways to add more color to your life:

- Go for a walk and notice the colors you are drawn to.
- Take a stroll in nature and see how many shades of green you can find.
- Pick wildflowers and place them in a small vase.
- Add a pop of color to your clothes or accessories.; pick colors that bring you joy.
- Add color to a room with a painting, a pillow, or a throw blanket.
- Eat colorful fruits and veggies, which are packed with nutrients.

Sometimes, we feel stuck in a gray existence. That's when we need to reset. Here's an exercise to help you rebalance the colors in your energy field:

- Shake your body out to help ground and center yourself.
- Rub your palms together to wake up the energy points there.
- Bring your palms to face each other as if you're holding a ball of bright, white light—white light contains all the colors in the color spectrum. Play with this ball of light; make it bigger or smaller, or rotate your hands around it.
- Next, gently bring the ball of light to your solar plexus, which is at the top of your abdomen, just under your breastbone. Feel the ball's light spread from your solar plexus throughout your body.
- You could also imagine the white light emanating from your hands to wherever it's needed. Give it a few minutes. Breathe in the light.

Try this exercise with a focus on each color of the rainbow: red, orange, yellow, green, blue, indigo, and violet. Some colors may feel easier to work with than others; that's okay. Breathe in each color daily to get used to them all.

Praying for Others and Group Prayer

Prayer is simply talking to the Universe, stating and sending your conscious intentions through spirit's wireless network straight to the Divine. Journalist and author Lynn McTaggart has spent years studying intention and learned that a healing intention benefits both the receiver and sender of an intention. In other words, when you pray for others, it helps you, too. Studies show that people praying for others feel a greater sense of oneness and inner peace than those who pray only for themselves—and praying with a group amplifies these effects.

Check this out for yourself. Say a prayer for others. Incorporate the suggestions below to ramp up the power of your prayer, and remember that your thoughts become a prayer when you're sincere.

- Meditate before you pray to align your mind, body, and spirit. Prayer is not just about thoughts but also alignment and connection. (You could use the Opening and Centering the Heart Field exercise in Part 1.)

- When you need to pray for yourself, pray for others as well. When we give, we also receive.

- Ask for the answer to your prayer to benefit "the good of all." Also, allow the answer to be what you desire or "something better"; this way, you leave room for the miracles you can't imagine.

- Feel gratitude for your prayers being received.

- Trust that what's best will unfold in divine timing.

Here's an example of a prayer I use:

Dear Universe,

Thank you for this opportunity to heal myself by helping others. I ask that everyone receive a healing of body, mind, and spirit. Please raise everyone's vibration here so we can notice and be open to the everyday miracles and love all around us. There is more than enough love to go around because Your love, and therefore our love, is infinite. Please help everyone in this group release their worries to the Divine and trust that all is well. I ask for this or better for the good of all. Thank you, thank you, thank you. I love you, I love you, I love you.

As Edgar Cayce said, "Why worry when you can pray?" Trust in Spirit and the power of your prayer, and take steps aligned with your prayer.

A Double Embrace

A double embrace is helpful anytime you need a hug. Whether you're feeling down, overwhelmed, or need to ground yourself, give yourself a cocoon to rest in and rebalance your energy. Here's how you can soothe yourself with a double embrace (Peter Levine's work on trauma and somatic release inspired the first part of this exercise):

1. Take your right hand and wrap it around your left chest, by your heart.

2. Then, wrap your left hand around your right arm and feel your heart and breath. Doing this brings your awareness to your physical body and its rhythms.

3. Next, add the spirit dimension to your embrace with an angelic embrace—it doesn't matter whether you believe in angels. Imagine an angel, maybe your guardian angel, enveloping you with angel wings, helping you feel safe and secure in a loving embrace.

You are always supported, especially during the difficult times. Let yourself feel that.

The Pink Eraser Meditation

One night, my whole family watched the movie *Stargirl*, and lo and behold, it inspired this unexpected gem of a meditation. It is a simple yet profound way to get to know your essence.

1. Imagine a big pink eraser (actually hold one if you have trouble visualizing this), and pretend you're erasing your physical body, from your toes to the top of your head.

2. When you're done, you'll be left with your essence: this is you. You are a spirit that is presently embodied in this human experience, and you can see, hear, and be in this state of pure universal knowing, love, and oneness.

3. If you desire to go deeper, ask yourself who you are without your home, your job, your past, etc. Can you get

a sense of your essence? You can create in the world from this loving core.

I have a friend whose son has cerebral palsy. He has difficulty controlling his movements, but his mind is intact. Once, he asked his dad, "I know this [pointing to his body] is not me. So, where am I?" He knew that despite his body's limitations, his spirit was limitless. We can reflect and connect with our inner light when we're not moving around and busy doing. And when we're in touch with our true nature—love—we will naturally make decisions that nourish ourselves and our planet.

Angel Tea Meditation

In this meditation, you can ask specific beings for guidance, whether someone who's crossed over, the angels, or other loving guides. You could also ask people you admire, deceased or alive, if they could mentor you. Because you're communicating via spirit, there are no limits to what you can do in this meditation. Everything, whether in the physical world or intangible dimensions, is part of the Oneness. Go ahead and gather a team of loving beings to help you in various ways. Spiritual teacher and author Lorna Byrne says many "unemployed angels" are just waiting for us to ask them for help. So, why not invite the angels for tea?

1. Imagine you're sitting at a round table or having a picnic with an angel or a host of angels. Don't worry if it seems like you're making this all up—exercise your imagination.

2. Ask questions and have a conversation. I get some of my best ideas this way.

3. When you're ready to end the tea party, thank the angels. Consider setting up a regular tea time with them.

How to Do Nothing

My tai chi instructor told me a story about a tai chi master who was so adept at nonresistance that a bird resting on his palm could not lift off. The bird needed to push off to take flight, but the master provided no resistance to the bird's push. Tai chi masters are "masters" because of their nonresistance. If you try to push a tai chi master over, they will move out of the way, and you'll likely lose your balance and fall.

Such mastery of nonresistance reminds me of Lao Tzu's teaching, "Do nothing, and all is done." It's a paradox that "doing nothing" can feel difficult yet require no effort at the same time. When we no longer resist life, we step into the ease of living. Here's a practice to cultivate nonresistance:

1. Start with a big breath, inhaling through the nose and slowly exhaling through the mouth. You can even make an "ah" sound as you exhale.

2. Shake out your arms, legs, and the rest of your body.

3. Take a few slow, deep breaths to help you settle in. When you inhale, breathe in love; when you exhale, let go of what no longer serves you.

4. Now, with loving awareness, notice the thoughts, feelings, and sensations that come up.

5. When "issues" arise, ask yourself how you can approach the issue in the most loving way possible. What would you do if you were only love? What would you do if you knew everything would work out for the good of all? And how can you love yourself through everything?

6. Love will guide you on the path of nonresistance because, as *A Course in Miracles* teaches, everything is love or a call for love.

7. How can you love more? Start by loving yourself, and you'll have a wellspring of infinite love for others.

PART IV

The Intuitive Human

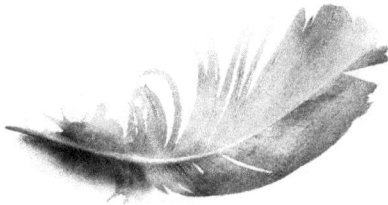

You are not just a body, a mind, or a spirit. Human beings are all three, and Divinity is in every part. Spirit brings the light and love, igniting your mind and thoughts to create a full sensory experience in the body. We need all dimensions—body, mind, and spirit—to be in harmony for us to feel whole.

Our thoughts, actions, feelings, and being matter; they send unique patterns of vibrations into the world and beyond in a ripple effect. We all have an impact on the world around us. We are dreaming the world together, each of us a unique thread in the tapestry of the Universe. Your life is an expression of the Oneness, and you can consciously co-create your life with the Oneness. American transcendentalist Henry David Thoreau said, "Our truest life is when we are in dreams awake."

In this book's final two chapters, we will pull it all together. It's time to dream and play!

CHAPTER 10

THE ART OF INTUITIVE LIVING

"Health is in the flow."

W hen I was five, I was fascinated by a dried-up old stump in the back of the playground. I would trace its jagged edges with my eyes, following the little peaks and valleys. I figured the tree must have fallen on its own because there wasn't a clear cut. The stump's rough surface was beautiful to me. I pretended it was a map of my world. I would scoop up the fine gray dirt and sprinkle it like fairy dust over the stump, imagining the world however I dreamed it to be. I don't remember why I thought to do that, but I do remember what I hoped to feel—wonder, peace, and happiness.

My young self still inspires me to remember that in this chaotic world of jagged edges and infinite beauty, we can create what we'd like together, and we start at the core of our *being*:

The role of the spirit is to BE.

The role of the mind is to CREATE.

The role of the body is to FEEL.

The role of our being is to LOVE.

The Importance of Play

What is play? Dr. Stuart Brown is a psychiatrist who founded the National Institute of Play. This is his definition of play: "a state of mind that one has when absorbed in an activity that provides enjoyment and a suspension of the sense of time. And play is self-motivated, so you want to do it again and again."[1] We play for the sake of play because it's fun, he tells us. Play doesn't have to have a purpose other than to bring joy.

Do you remember how you played when you were in kindergarten? The American Academy of Pediatrics encourages pediatricians to prescribe play to children, their parents, and caregivers. The National Institute of Play has been studying the effects of play on children and adults for several decades. Here's an overview of the benefits they've identified:

Table 15 - The Benefits of Play

BENEFITS	CHILDREN	ADULTS
Emotional processing	In play, children can act out scary or stressful situations and gain a sense of control. It's common to see them play a scene over and over again. Each time is an opportunity to process intense emotions. Play helps children develop self-awareness and emotional regulation.	Adults continue to develop self-awareness from the feedback of play, while the flow of play helps to release tension and stress. Whether adults appreciate play or are themselves playing, play provides safe opportunities to experience intense emotions, and rising up to play after a life challenge fosters resilience and optimism.
Cognition	Play provides opportunities to learn through experience—the best type of learning. Children interact with their environment, experiment with their imagination, and gain problem-solving skills in play.	Learning is lifelong. Adults who embrace learning exercise a diverse network of neural pathways that improve fluid thinking and memory.

Table 15 - The Benefits of Play *(continued)*

BENEFITS	CHILDREN	ADULTS
Perseverance	The self-motivation in play encourages learning and mastery. Children learn to flow with the ups and downs when learning is fun.	The self-motivation in play encourages learning and mastery. Adults learn to flow with the ups and downs when learning is fun.
Communication	In play, children practice their language and social skills, using what they learn from each other and the adults in their lives.	Play involves interacting with ourselves, each other, and the world and provides ways to express the soul, whether through words, movement, drama, music, color, etc.
Connection	During play, bonds that transcend differences are established, and children develop friendships.	Play is a way for adults to get along and can encourage more empathy, compassion, trust, and intimacy.
Physical health	Active play promotes movement and develops strength and coordination.	Both active and creative play boosts the immune system, decreases cardiovascular risks, and builds strength and coordination.
Creativity	The imagination has no limits. The creativity of play honors the potential in each child to be anything they dream to be and to create anything they desire to make.	We are limitless beings with an infinite imagination. We can dream and transform physical reality because of our dreams. Play fosters curiosity, innovation, and problem-solving.

Play's Personalities

What do you do for fun? What did you do for fun when you were little? What would you do if you had all the time and money in the world?

You're the one who gets to choose what is fun, and it doesn't have to follow logic. Sometimes, people aren't sure what's fun for them anymore; they've lost touch because of all the busyness in life.

That National Institute of Play's founder, Stuart Brown, has come up with eight "play personalities" based on decades of interviews.[2] Although these archetypes are not driven by scientific data per se, Dr. Brown has found they help people identify what inherently motivates them. You don't have to fit into only one category from the following list, though one may be more prominent. We can be drawn to a few types, and how we play can also vary in different situations.

Table 16 – Eight Play Personalities

Collector	Collectors find particular objects or experiences intriguing, such as collecting shells, cars, wine, art, books, etc.
Competitor	Competitors love the thrill of a game and keeping score, whether participating or watching. Competitive sports fall into this category.
Creator or Artist	There's an artist in each of us. We are all meant to create, whether through a recognized art form, a business endeavor, or some other creative expression.
Director	Directors love organizing and planning ways to unite people, such as parties and other events.
Explorer	For explorers, the world is a playground of exploration, with physical places to explore as well as emotions and new perspectives.
Joker	The joker enjoys laughter and fun, whether clowning around, telling jokes, or pulling pranks.
Kinesthete	Kinesthetes have a hard time sitting still because they need to move. Movement helps them think. They may play sports, practice martial arts, do yoga, exercise regularly, or enjoy dance. The emphasis for the kinesthete is on movement, not competition as it is for the competitor.
Storyteller	Storytellers enjoy playing with the imagination; they are writers, performers, and those who enjoy reading, movies, and shows.

You are unique, and you can bring any of these play personalities into different aspects of your life. The world needs you to play, create, and share what you love in your unique way.

Embracing the Opportunities in Failure

The soul desires to love. The act of creating is one way we express our love, and since it is also a form of play, creating provides all of the benefits of play, particularly helping us process difficult emotions, connect with ourselves and others, deepen our intuition, and think innovatively. Inevitably, only some of our creations will work out as we hope. Sometimes, what we make will fall apart. Think of a child playing with blocks or building a sandcastle; ideally, like a child, when our creation falls apart, we begin again because we enjoy creating. This response characterizes the growth mindset we discussed in chapter 5. When whatever we've created doesn't work out, we have an opportunity to grow through failure. Give yourself permission to fail because you're going to mess up sometimes—we all do—and it's okay.

In 2020, I gathered with over two dozen artists in a virtual conference to discuss art and healing. One of those artists, Travis Carr, is the local high school ceramics teacher and a friend of mine. Here's what he had to say about pottery, failure, and resilience:

"So many people beat themselves up for every little thing that they do. They suffer from anxiety and social pressures, and kids deal with social media these days. I think it's important for them to feel good about something they make. Ceramics is a medium where you have to learn how to fail and be okay with it. So many times you'll make this thing that you're so proud of, and it might blow up in the kiln, or it might make it through, but then you glaze it, and the glaze gets ruined, and you have to start over—and you have to be okay with it. One of my students was a salutatorian, and her entire speech was about ceramics and sculpture and her experience with art. She talked about embracing failure—taking that object and creating something beautiful with it, whether from the object itself or the experience, and moving forward from it. I think that's something that's needed right now: the ability to accept failure, put a positive spin on it, and move forward to create something beautiful from that experience."

Travis's point about ceramics teaching people how to meet failure touches on a valuable lesson. We all have a remarkable capacity for resilience. Like the natural world, we find a way to grow, change, and recover. That's why we have a built-in trauma-release mechanism. We've made plenty of mistakes individually and collectively as humans. Now is our time to learn from our failures, bounce back, and shine a light in any darkness.

Shine Your Light

Even in life's messiness, there is beauty. You and your inner light are a part of that beauty. Your light is always there, even if it seems eclipsed at times. How can you access your light at any moment, even when life is hard? Here are a few suggestions:

- Sit in the stillness. When life feels chaotic, it helps to get very quiet and rest in the stillness. Without the outside world's distractions, you can tap into the loving and encouraging guidance inside you.

- Help someone. The more love we give, the more we have, and the more it grows. Fred Rogers of *Mister Roger's Neighborhood* taught us: "In times of trouble, look for the helpers." You can be one of the helpers.

- Gaze at a sunrise or a sunset. There's a reason we're drawn to sunrises and sunsets: the sun's light reminds us of the light in our hearts.

- Study the patterns and qualities of a flower. Consider how a bud becomes a flower and can't become anything other than itself. Engage all your senses to enjoy the flower's beauty. The feelings a flower evokes can illuminate the light in your heart.

- Add laughter. We are all children of the Divine. See if you can find at least one thing to smile, laugh, or giggle about each day. Warm-hearted humor and laughter can uplift any moment.

Everything Can Be an Art

The art of living involves you being you. When your authenticity and purpose are aligned, there's this marvelous effect: they become one.

When authenticity and purpose are unaligned, people feel they must "find themselves" or "their purpose." Do you see how authenticity and purpose are actually one? Love is the power that makes them one.

Remember this?

Love *(awareness of the soul)* + **Intention** *(purposeful thought)*
= **Creation** *(the soul's loving expression)*

Every movement has meaning when we're in creation's flow because it expresses the soul moving through us. Artists are aware of this. Travis Carr, whom we heard from earlier, says that in ceramics: "Every mark is purposeful. When you look at the final dried and glazed ceramic, you can see every impression made on that clay." Mark Hopper is a master blacksmith who can look at a piece of metalwork and see the story and thought process of the blacksmith who made it.

When your authenticity, purpose, thoughts, words, and actions are in harmony with the Creative Forces, anything in life can become an art. We are in a state of flow—truer expressions of Light (Divine guidance, soul wisdom, intuition) and Love (consciousness, soul awareness). We bring beauty and color (expressions of Light) into our human experience, and our Love and Understanding help us feel safe to be who we are. This is truly living.

Let's add Light to our equation of understanding:

Love *(awareness of the soul)* + **Light** *(Divine guidance)*
+ **Intention** *(purposeful thought)*
= **The Art of Intuitive Living** *(conscious co-creation)*

You can bring conscious intention and purpose to anything you do. For example, when you give to someone, you can be aware of the love you're sharing with them. You can be love as well as feel, know, think, speak, and act with love. This love starts with love for yourself, and when you can allow yourself to be authentic, you can allow others to be authentic. This state of being is so liberating! You do not need to be the hero or the victim. It feels good to contribute to another's happiness, but even better when you don't need to control their response.

Here's what conscious giving to another might look like in your everyday life:

- Share tea or a meal. When you give someone a cup of tea or share a meal, do it with the intention to nourish and love them.

- Give a gift. When you give a gift, feel your love and joy for the other person and yourself. How someone receives what you give matters less than how you feel when giving. Since you are not a hero or a victim, everyone is free to be as they are.

- Send a loving note, text, or email. Your words are powerful and have a direct impact on you and others. What words will convey your love and respect for another and yourself?

- Go for a walk and bless what you see. Wherever you place your loving awareness—the trees, the sky, the other beings there—honor the focus of your attention with love and light, and wherever you walk, imagine you're leaving behind a trail of sunshine.

When we remember we are part of the Oneness, it's easy to see that helping another is also helping ourselves and that taking care of ourselves is also taking care of others. Similarly, when we're down, we bring others down with us, and when we degrade others, we also degrade ourselves. The more we live in love, the more we will see what's true in ourselves and others, and the more thankful we'll be for what's true. This is the art of living.

Living in Gratitude

Gratitude instantaneously elevates our experience. It helps us get through life's messiness and keeps us going. Our souls have always known the importance of gratitude. Now, research from the field of positive psychology is backing up what our souls know: gratitude and happiness are connected. Gratitude is one of the most powerful ways to collaborate with the Oneness and consciously co-create our lives. When we choose to be thankful, we steer our life toward more joy.

Understanding key aspects of gratitude can help you appreciate its value to you.

- Gratitude plays a role in your ability to flow with life.
- Like giving love, the more you give thanks, the more

thankful you feel. It's a moment-to-moment practice, just like love and kindness.

- Gratitude for your dreams, hopes, and desires, even before they manifest, creates a vibration that magnetizes your dreams, hopes, and desires to you.

This meditation can help you experience the magnificence of gratitude:

1. Imagine you are in a universe of abundance with no time or space. There is enough for your hopes, dreams, and desires and everyone else's hopes, dreams, and desires.

2. Imagine how you would feel if your dreams had already come true, or imagine your best day ever. What would you feel, see, hear, and sense? Play it out in your imagination like a movie.

3. Let yourself feel how thankful you would be to live fully. Feeling gratitude supercharges your energy field so that you *become* the vibration of your dreams and magnetize them. The magnetic effect comes from the vibrancy of your soul.

4. Take the steps necessary to actualize and live your dreams when you're not meditating. Keep in mind that the Universe may guide you in unexpected ways. Trust the process. How your hopes, dreams, and desires unfold may not happen as you imagine.

When applying for a residency in pediatrics, I didn't get into my top choice—but the Universe sorted things out for me better than I could have imagined. I had always wanted to live in New York City at some point in my life, preferably before having kids. I didn't think it would happen, though. When I was applying for residencies, too many practical reasons worked against it. New York City was too expensive, I wasn't familiar with its medical programs, I was getting married, and my fiancé didn't have a job in New York. So, I applied to programs in other cities.

When I got the dreaded phone call and learned that I didn't get into any of the programs I applied to, there were tears, embarrassment, and panic. What was I going to do? What was my fiancé going to do? Had I messed up our lives? After a meeting with my medical school, we found a residency for me—in the Bronx, a borough of New York City! The impractical suddenly became practical, the rejection became an opportunity, and the perceived limitation was a redirect to other possibilities. As the Universe would have it, my fiancé's employer easily transferred him to a position in Manhattan. Living in New York, I discovered yoga, meditation, and integrative medicine, and my husband and I enjoyed an amazing set of friends. I am forever grateful.

Living in gratitude is saying "yes!" to the life of your dreams. When we choose gratitude, we step into the flow of living. Life can open up in ways better than we might have imagined.

Letting Your Life Force Flow

When your body, mind, and spirit are aligned and grounded, the Universe can freely flow through you. The mind aligns with guidance from the Universe, and the body becomes an energy channel for conscious manifestation. Seven major energy centers are arranged along the central line of your body. They are called *chakras* in Sanskrit. The central energy channel runs from the pubic bone to the crown of the head. In osteopathy, we refer to this channel as one of the "midlines" of the body. In acupuncture, it is called the "central meridian." The major endocrine glands are also located along the midline; bundles of nerves known as "nerve plexi" correspond to the various chakras, or energy centers.

In the yoga tradition, the energy that travels up the midline is called "kundalini energy." Kundalini energy, which is the life force, travels along the midline, connects the major energy centers, and extends the energy from the midline to the rest of your body. (See Figure 9 on the next page.) When your life force can flow freely, you feel fully alive, which is vital for conscious creation. When the midline's energy centers are open, you have more energy, trust yourself more, access your intuition more easily, feel more confident, flow with life, experience more joy, connect with others more easily, and manifest consciously. Your heart-centered creations give Spirit a tangible expression in physical form. When the midline energy centers are open and the kundalini energy is flowing, you can purposefully create your life story.

I often tell my patients, "Health is in the flow." Flow is essential for so many aspects of living, from the flow of blood, to the flow of emotions, to the flow of life transitions. Beth was a patient who had ongoing post-viral symptoms: fatigue, headaches, neck pain, ringing

Figure 9 - Kundalini Energy Traveling up the Midline

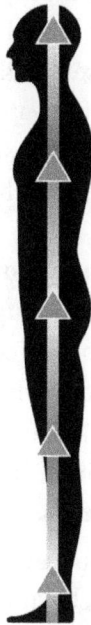

in the ears, painful periods, and worsening seasonal allergies. I worked with her to help reset the nervous system, release tension in the body, uncurl the heart, and open up the midline. We did this through cranial osteopathic treatment, homeopathic remedies, and exercises I had her do at home (all included in this book). In less than two months, most of her physical symptoms had resolved, and Beth's husband, a professional counselor, noticed a dramatic shift in her that he said was equal to years of counseling.

To open up Beth's midline, I walked her through this exercise. First, I asked her to notice any *physical tension* in her sacral pelvic area. Then, I asked her to breathe into that tension without any goal or agenda. She was simply to notice and breathe. Within a few minutes, she felt a softening, a slight relaxation, in the area. Next, I asked her to notice any *emotional tension* in the sacral pelvic area. Again, Beth was to notice what came up, nothing more. She didn't have to look for an emotion; she just had to notice whatever surfaced, and the emotions didn't have to make sense. Within a few minutes, Beth noticed her lower back easing up and her pelvis releasing more tension. Then,

I asked her to notice the space between all the cells, atoms, and tissues in her sacral pelvic area. We are mostly space, after all! I asked her to breathe into the space, allowing her soul to ground and fully inhabit her body. For a third time, Beth relaxed in the sacral pelvic area. She could also breathe better. At the end of the appointment, Beth was beaming. She said she felt more expanded and a sense of freedom and joy in her body, mind, and spirit. I could see that her midline was glowing.

Exercise: Letting the Life Force Flow

This is the exercise I walked Beth through for you to use. It is a breathing and mindfulness meditation that connects your body, mind, and spirit. Choose an area of your body where you feel tension or discomfort. The area does not have to have obvious pain; for example, you might feel a weight on your chest, heaviness in your shoulders, or tightness in your abdomen or pelvis.

1. Bring a gentle, nonjudgmental awareness to the area of tension in your physical body. Then, breathe into that tension without a goal or agenda. Simply notice and breathe for a few minutes. The physical tension might feel the same, or you might feel a softening or a slight release. There is no right or wrong to whatever you experience and no judgment on whether there is a change.

2. Next, notice any emotional tension in the same area. You don't have to look for any emotions—just notice whatever surfaces. There might be a primary emotion or a jumble of emotions; the emotion(s) don't have to make sense. Notice with gentle awareness. Again, there's no right or wrong answer. Then, breathe into the emotional tension without a goal or agenda. Any emotion that surfaces is allowed to be as it is. Continue to breathe into whatever arises for several minutes. After some moments, the emotional tension might be the same, or you might notice a softening or a relaxation. Whatever you notice is okay. There is no goal.

3. Now, bring your gentle awareness to the space between the cells, atoms, and tissues. That space has so much potential because it's part of the Stillness, the source from which all things arise. Your pure essence—your unique emanation of the Stillness— can also be more easily perceived in this space. Breathe into the space, letting your whole being feel its vibrance, expansiveness,

and welcoming of your soul. You might feel this as a lightening or expansion in your body and biofield. Whether or not you feel this, your breath and awareness *are* helping you integrate body, mind, and spirit.

Intuitive Being

It's time to wake up to who you are. You are light. You are love. You are stardust—literally. You are an intuitive being; this is your nature. The more you get to know yourself, the more you'll step into your intuitive superpowers. You don't have to wait. You can open any page of this book and find ways to access your intuition.

As we discussed in Part 2, the ultimate statement of divine creation is "I AM." The vibration of "I AM" is the primordial sound of creation. "I AM" is the most conscious way to be in the world. When said with love and sincerity, statements that begin with "I AM" will help open the midline and your creative energy. When you say, think, and feel "I AM" statements from the light and love of your being, then you harmonize with the Universal Oneness, and the vibrations of "I AM" flow up your midline, through your heart center, your throat chakra, continuing to illuminate your mind, eyes, crown, and entire energy field. You might feel the energy circulating around you and flowing back up the midline again. You are a miraculous being—remember that.

Figure 10 - Creation Energy Circulating in a Torus Shape

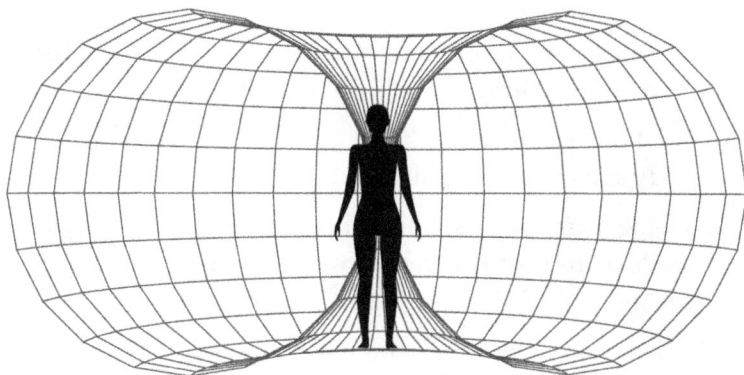

This figure represents a cross-section of the torus-shaped field emanating from each of us.

I am closing this chapter with three "I AM" statements that will support you to be who you already are:

I AM INTUITIVE

I AM CREATIVE

I AM LOVE

Believe in yourself. I believe in you.

Summary

The art of living involves fully expressing of your being—your body, mind, and spirit. You express your love in the world through creation. Creation is an art, and in that sense, life is also an art—it is the art of being ourselves.

1. Play helps you get into a flow state, where you feel at ease with yourself and can live out your potential.

2. Play helps with emotional processing, perseverance, cognition, communication, connection, physical health, and creativity.

3. Explore your play personality(ies) using the eight play personalities Dr. Stuart Brown identified: the collector, the competitor, the creator or artist, the director, the explorer, the joker, the kinesthete, and the storyteller.

4. There is only one you, which means there is no competition.

5. When you embrace failure, you can create something else from it, something new and even beautiful.

6. Anything you do in life becomes an art when your authenticity and purpose are aligned.

7. Living in gratitude will help you get through life's messiness while motivating you to keep going. Living in gratitude is saying "yes!" to living your best life.

8. When your body, mind, and spirit are aligned and grounded, life can flow freely through you.

Life has so much more meaning when we live from the heart. We feel more vibrant and alive when we express our soul's love. Health is in the flow. When you live from your heart, you can see that problems show you where a healthy flow needs to be re-established. Every area of your life is part of your intuitive compass.

CHAPTER 11

MULTIDIMENSIONAL MEDICINE

*"A healthcare system guided by love and
compassion that provides more people access to
deeper healing using fewer resources is possible."*

We've neglected certain aspects of our health within modern medicine for far too long, and we can look to the history of medicine to explain why. During the sixteenth and seventeenth centuries, advances in science led to a separation in studies of the body, mind, and spirit. Medicine and healthcare focused on the body, while religion claimed our relationship to Spirit. Then, later in the nineteenth century, psychology emerged as a study of the mind and behavior. When we separate the body from the mind and the spirit, we limit our understanding of the depth of healing possible when we bring all three together, which were never meant to be separated in the first place.

It's not that science is wrong. Instead, it's that our scientific understanding is incomplete. The universe is so vast we can't know it all right now, so we must approach the mind, body, and spirit with the understanding that our knowledge is incomplete. We must also approach science with the respectful knowing that our scientific understanding is likewise incomplete.

I use the term "multidimensional medicine" to emphasize the many dimensions of our being and the expanded perspectives of our intuition. As we discussed at the beginning of this book, intuition is that spark of inner guidance that comes through your body, mind, and spirit, and it is always loving, supportive, and encouraging. In other words, deep down—maybe deep, deep down—your being knows how to heal.

All Healing Begins with Love

All healing has one Source, and all healing is Love. When we love, we also remember that we *are* love. The more you love and understand yourself, the more vibrant and alive your being feels. The magnificent vibration of love emanates outwards and all around you like a wave. Those love waves inspire other people, helping them heal as well.

That's how I feel in my practice: I couldn't help people the way I do if I didn't love them. When you love yourself and another being, it's much easier to understand the other. The heart connection helps to expand what you're able to perceive. I feel it's my job as a physician to see the light and love within you—your true source of health. Regardless of where you came from, your walk of life, or what you've done, the light of life within you cannot be undone. It's the part of you that will continue after the physical ends. Yes, sometimes when you don't feel quite right and have symptoms of illness or feel "off," it may feel covered up, but the light is still there. I love to help people see their light and align with it to realize their limitless potential in Love and Oneness.

During the early years of my practice, I remember seeing a mom in the waiting room who was distraught because her daughter was having an allergic reaction to dairy. She had not eaten any dairy; the reaction was simply from her contact with dairy. This mom had tears in her eyes from the stress and worry. I guess the concern on my face matched hers because Emily told me my response touched her. She said it was the most caring response she felt from a physician. That struck me because I didn't feel I had done anything other than stay present with her while she told me their story.

All healing must begin with love. The process of helping is then an expression of that love. Remember the patient Doris I told you about in the introduction? She had been hospitalized with pneumonia and revealed for the first time that she had been sexually abused. We didn't know what to do with her trauma, so we ignored it. But had we approached her with love, love would have guided us in what to do. The first step would have been to show Doris she mattered by acknowledging her with loving-kindness. Why would physicians be any other way?

A Healthcare Culture of Compassion and Kindness

The culture of healthcare and medicine needs to shift toward more compassion and kindness for both self and others. Does that sound silly? Or too obvious to talk about? I would have thought so before medical school. During my years of training, I witnessed a cut-throat and competitive culture. I saw how easily students and residents were put down and not treated as equal human beings. Looking back, it's also easy for me to see how tired and stressed most people were. Often the stakes were high as we dealt with life-and-death decisions. But life-and-death decisions are best made when we're feeling our best, and kindness and compassion come easily. This is not only common sense but also backed by studies that show fatigue and distress are associated with medical errors.[1]

Kindness and happiness also go hand in hand. When we're kind to people, we're happier, and when we're happy, we're kinder to people.[2] Acts of kindness also affect the chemical and hormone production in the body.[3] Kindness boosts oxytocin (the love hormone), substance P (an endorphin-like chemical that decreases pain), dopamine (a neurotransmitter of joy), and serotonin (a good-mood neurotransmitter). Neurosurgeon Dr. James Doty, a professor at Stanford University and the founder and director of the Center for Compassion and Altruism Research and Education, has found that when health care is delivered with kindness, people get better faster.

Fortunately, a movement of kindness is currently gaining momentum. The Greater Good Science Center at the University of California, Berkeley, "studies the psychology, sociology, and neuroscience of well-being and teaches skills that foster a thriving, resilient, and compassionate society."[4] Their work includes helping healthcare professionals boost their happiness to create a meaningful life and avoid burnout. Many other groups with this mission of supporting medical practitioners exist, and many continue to form both locally and globally. I keep a list of updated resources on this book's website: allworldspress.com.

Trauma-Informed Health Care

Despite research showing that stress and trauma can cause disease, our healthcare system is ill-equipped to address this relationship. Recall how a trauma response and release are a natural part of being human. When overwhelmed, however, the trauma response can get stuck, constantly releasing stress hormones and other chemicals when the original threat has passed. Chronic trauma patterns are then left to wreak havoc on all aspects of a person's health, including the nervous, immune, endocrine, and digestive systems, and their mental-emotional health. In neglecting the role of trauma on health, modern medicine has missed the mark. In some cases, the impact of trauma on illness is completely ignored, as it was with Doris. Think of the depth of healing Doris could have accessed if health care incorporated a trauma-informed mindset.

Fortunately, interest in understanding the impact of trauma and how we can aid ourselves and others in recovery is growing. Trauma researchers and other healthcare professionals are working to increase awareness throughout medicine and society in general. Renowned addiction specialist Dr. Gabor Mate has shed light on the connection between neglecting the burden of stress and the rise in chronic illnesses. Psychiatrist Bruce Perry has had many discussions with Oprah Winfrey on the neuroscientific explanations of the trauma response. He has coauthored a book with her on trauma, *What Happened to You? Conversations on Trauma, Resilience, and Healing.*

Trauma-informed healthcare professionals hope to normalize conversations about tender matters of the heart and promote healing. Imagine feeling safe to discuss how you feel without embarrassment or shame. Imagine your physician having a good understanding of how what you've been through is contributing to your current state of health. Imagine they can also help you navigate a path to recovery that includes addressing subconscious trauma patterns. Imagine trauma-informed health care as the new norm. All this starts by healing health care from within.

Healer, Heal Thyself

No one can work to their potential when their health is not up to par. Physicians and other healthcare workers must address their mental and physical health in an integrative health model. Every person is deserving of love and care. If you're in healthcare, you've got to walk the talk.

This was driven into me during my integrative medicine fellowship at the University of Arizona. It was so refreshing. I had never felt so cared for in my medical career. We ate fresh, healthy food at conferences and practiced tai chi together in the mornings. It was a far cry from the pharmaceutical-sponsored lunches of pizza or chicken and biscuits during my previous medical training. There was even a McDonald's on the first floor of my hospital in residency!

During medical school and residency, we rarely had any debriefing for the stress and traumas we regularly witnessed. We would see people die, and the accompanying stories were sometimes horrific. Colleagues also experienced their own personal crises, such as miscarriages or the sudden death of loved ones, and they'd have to return to work soon afterward. At the time, I wondered how to approach everyone who was hurting, not only from physical pain but also from obvious mental, emotional, and spiritual pain. These situations reminded me of the awkwardness and despair I felt with Doris. I hoped for more guidance, which brings me full circle to why I wrote this book.

To take medicine to the next level, healthcare professionals must care for themselves. We are human beings, too, and we need to treat ourselves with humanity. Otherwise, we will break down, and ultimately, the system will break down. And that's about where we are now. According to a 2019 study in the *Annals of Medicine*, doctor burnout was estimated to cost the US healthcare system roughly $4.6 billion a year—and that was before the 2020 pandemic.[5] A 2022 study published in *The Mayo Clinic Proceedings* reported that physician burnout had reached an all-time high of 63 percent, consistent across specialties.[6] Overall, healthcare costs show us that we aren't using our resources to the best of our abilities—but there is a more efficient way to spend less and help more.

Doing More with Less

"Doing more with less" was inventor and architect Buckminster Fuller's design slogan. He was ahead of his time. Bucky, as he was affectionately called, referred to our planet as Spaceship Earth. On a spaceship you have a certain amount of resources to keep the astronauts alive. In the same way, Earth has a certain amount of resources to keep its inhabitants alive. We have to use these resources with respect. Hence, Bucky's motto of doing more with less.

Health care can follow a similar philosophy. How can we use less and do more? How might we spend less while helping people be healthier? The present healthcare system is overwhelmed, and chronic diseases are skyrocketing. According to the Commonwealth Fund, in 2021, the United States had the worst healthcare system among 11 high-income countries—despite spending the most on healthcare![7]

We *can* heal our current healthcare system. We *can* help more people. It will require a paradigm shift from a disease-focused to a health-focused model. For example, let's consider our approach to high cholesterol and hypertension. In a disease-focused model, a physician writes a prescription to counter the illness, which is likely paid for by insurance. The physician has very little, if any, time to talk about a healthy diet, nor would the physician be paid to do so in this model. But in a health-focused model, a physician could write a prescription for healthy food, which would also be paid for by insurance. (They are doing this in Michigan with their "Prescriptions for Health" program!) he health-focused model affects a person's life more because you support their overall health. This approach sometimes reverses disease and can prevent downstream complications. It can improve a patient's mood, energy, sleep, and more, allowing the person to have a better quality of life and likely better relationships. This kind of system would drive down the cost of health care, making it more feasible to provide universal healthcare coverage.

Fortunately, there is hope as new models like this are being studied. Here's a sample from one such report out of Tufts University: "When the researchers ran their model with a prescription for fruits and vegetables, they estimated that 1.93 million cardiovascular events would be prevented and $39.7 billion would be saved. When they ran it with the broader prescription for healthy foods, they estimated that

3.28 million cardiovascular events and 120,000 diabetes cases would be avoided and $100.2 billion would be saved."[8]

There is enough for everyone *if* we create a system with that measure in mind. We can do more with less.

Finding a Holistic Physician

People often ask me how to find a physician with my philosophy, knowledge, and approach. Every practitioner is unique, and there are several variables to consider when deciding on a healthcare practitioner. No one practitioner has the same experience and training as another. Here are some factors to consider:

- **Character.** Is the physician warm, kind, compassionate, and loving? Do you feel at ease speaking with them? Do they have a nonjudgmental presence? Do you feel safe sharing vulnerable information with them? Are they leading by example with their self-care?

- **Knowledge and experience.** Does the physician have a foundational understanding of nutrition? Have they sought out training in integrative medicine or holistic studies? Do they give suggestions that extend beyond pharmaceutical prescriptions and supplements? Are they willing to investigate the least invasive options first?

- **Willingness to collaborate.** Is the physician willing to collaborate with other healthcare professionals? Are they willing to partner with you? Do they listen to your ideas? Can you ask your questions easily?

- **Honesty.** Is the practitioner willing to say "I don't know" when they're unsure? Do they have enough self-awareness to realize the limits of their knowledge and experience? Do they have an air of transparency?

- **Curiosity.** Does the practitioner show interest in amazing stories of healing? Are they a forever student willing to learn and grow? Are they willing to research extraordinary results and difficult cases?

- **Believes in you.** Does the physician believe in you and your ability to love and be loved? Do you feel they care about you?

Can they see the light of health—your inner light—always in you?

- **Where to look.** The following organizations share a health-focused approach to healthcare. They believe in the innate healing power within each person, see the whole human being, emphasize the practitioner-patient partnership, prioritize prevention first, acknowledge that optimal health involves many aspects of life, and appreciate the healing power of love.

  - The Andrew Weil Center for Integrative Medicine at the University of Arizona is my alma mater. According to Dr. Andrew Weil, often regarded as the father of integrative medicine: "Integrative Medicine (IM) is healing-oriented medicine that takes account of the whole person, including all aspects of lifestyle. It emphasizes the therapeutic relationship between practitioner and patient, is informed by evidence, and makes use of all appropriate therapies." You can find an integrative medicine fellow on their website: awcim.arizona.edu/about/alumni.html.

  - **The Osteopathic Cranial Academy** (OCA) is near and dear to my heart. I've been a part of this organization since 2008 and am currently a faculty member. Dr. Weil is a huge fan of osteopathy, as was Edgar Cayce. The father of osteopathy, Dr. A. T. Still, said, "To find health should be the object of the doctor. Anyone can find disease." I hope more people learn about osteopathy, particularly cranial osteopathy. Osteopathy helps you tap into your innate health by restoring the natural flow and balance of energy within you. You can find a cranial osteopath on the academy's website: cranialacademy.org/find-a-physician/.

  - **The Academy of Integrative Health and Medicine** (AIHM) "is an interprofessional community of healthcare providers, researchers, and academics united by the shared value of treating the whole person—mind, body, spirit, community, and planet." The organization unifies "the diverse voices of traditional, complementary, and integrative health." The AIHM was formed in 1977 and has evolved over the decades. You can find an AIHM provider on their website: aihm.org/members/find-a-provider/.

If you can't find a physician near you with these qualities, consider supplementing visits to your regular physician with other healthcare practitioners, such as functional medicine practitioners, naturopaths, homeopaths, holistic nurses, trained herbalists, acupuncturists, Traditional Chinese Medicine professionals, Ayurvedic practitioners, energy medicine practitioners, chiropractors and other bodyworkers. Keep in mind that how nonmedical professions are regulated will vary from state to state and from country to country. Also, keep in mind the wide variation in styles among practitioners practicing the same modality. You will have your individual preference. Listen to your intuition when choosing!

Summary

We discussed the need and hope for a new wave of medicine, a healthcare system guided by love and compassion that aims to provide more people access to deeper healing using fewer resources. It *is* possible.

- We need to reintegrate mind, body, and spirit in health care.

- All healing begins with love.

- To change the current healthcare system, we need to prioritize a medical culture of loving-kindness.

- Because stress and trauma can cause disease, trauma-informed care is imperative to access deeper healing.

- Healer, heal thyself! Healthcare professionals must practice self-care.

- There is enough for everyone. Like Buckminster Fuller said, we can design with the intention of "doing more with less."

- We need to shift from a disease-focused approach in medicine to a health-focused approach.

- When looking for a health-focused physician, consider their character, knowledge and experience, willingness to collaborate, honesty, curiosity, and whether they believe in you.

* * *

Thank you for reading this book and joining me on this incredible journey. I hope you've found many gems to help you

- *Trust* yourself more

- *Feel* more connected to the Oneness

- *Hope* for a more harmonious future

- *Love* yourself, others, and the world around us more, and

- *Experience the beauty of living fully.*

If this book helps you and you have stories to share with me, I would love to hear from you!

You can connect with me at **welcome@allworldspress.com.**

Appendix:
Trauma Release Resources

- **Brainspotting** is a treatment in which the therapist uses a person's visual field to access unprocessed trauma. You can learn more and find providers at **brainspotting.com**.

- **Emotional Freedom Technique** is a mind-body technique that involves tapping on acupressure points to help resolve personal fears and trauma. It's also known as "tapping." Among the many resources available on EFT are founder Gary Craig's website, **emofree.com**, and Jessica and Nick Ortner's website, **thetappingsolution.com**.

- **Eye Movement Desensitization and Reprocessing**, also known as EMDR, is a psychotherapy treatment that alleviates the distress of disturbing life experiences and traumatic memories. You can learn more and find providers at **emdr.com**.

- **Tension & Trauma Releasing Exercises (TRE®)** were created by Dr. David Berceli, an international expert in trauma intervention and conflict resolution. You can learn more about these exercises and find providers at **traumaprevention.com**.

- **Bessel van der Kolk, MD,** has spent his career studying how children and adults adapt to traumatic experiences. His book on understanding and treating traumatic stress, *The Body Keeps the Score,* is a New York Times bestseller and has been published in 43 languages. You can learn more at **besselvanderkolk.com**.

- **Peter Levine, PhD,** is the developer of **Somatic Experiencing®**, a naturalistic and neurobiological approach to healing trauma. He is the author of several bestselling books on trauma, including *Waking the Tiger, Healing Trauma,* published in thirty languages. You can learn more at **somaticexperiencing.com**.

- **Gabor Maté , MD,** is a Canadian physician with a background in family practice and childhood development, with a special interest in trauma and its potential lifelong impacts on physical and mental health. His book *The Myth of Normal: Trauma, Illness & Healing in a Toxic Culture* examines how Western medicine's neglect of the trauma, stress, and pressures of modern-day living is connected to the upsurge in chronic illness and general ill health we are seeing today. You can learn more at **drgabormate.com.**

- **Bruce Perry, MD,** is a clinician, researcher , and professor in children's mental health and the neurosciences. His most recent book, *What Happened to You? Conversations on Trauma, Resilience, and Healing,* coauthored with Oprah Winfrey, explores a subtle but profound shift in approaching trauma that opens the door to resilience and healing in a proven and powerful way. You can learn more at **bdperry.com.**

RECOMMENDED RESOURCES

All Worlds Press is a publishing company dedicated to publishing and distributing wellness books of enlightenment. It is part of the **All Worlds Health** family, which includes Dr. Dijamco's integrative medical practice and the nonprofit All Worlds Foundation. *I AM Intuitive: A MultiDimensional Guide to Embrace Your Inner Light,* is the first book offered by All Worlds Press. To access the multimedia **bonus materials** for this book, including **additional graphics, dietary handouts, video demonstrations, and audio meditations** go to **allworldspress.com.**

Sheri Baker is the director of the Gary Craig Official EFT Training Center for the United States and other English-speaking countries. She also teaches an online study program, "Tapping Into the Truth," that integrates the **Emotional Freedom Technique** (EFT) with *A Course in Miracles.* You can learn more about Sheri and her services at **sheribaker.com.**

Richard Bartlett, DC, ND, is a chiropractor and naturopath with extraordinary healing abilities. He developed **Matrix Energetics** and the **Institute for Harmonic Resonance** to help people tap into conscious technology and their healing potential. You can learn more and sign up for online or in-person events at **i-hrt.com.**

The Book of Joy: Lasting Happiness in a Changing World is a conversation between the **Dalai Lama** and **Archbishop Desmond Tutu,** two great spiritual masters who are Nobel Prize recipients.

Brene´ Brown is a researcher and storyteller who has spent two decades studying courage, vulnerability, shame, and empathy. She is author of six *New York Times* bestselling books, including ***The Gifts of Imperfection, Daring Greatly***, and ***Rising Strong***. She is also the host of the podcasts ***Unlocking Us*** and ***Dare to Lead***. You can learn more at **brenebrown.com**.

Dr. Stuart Brown is a psychiatrist and founder of the **National Institute for Play** (NIFP). After decades of research on play, he is convinced that we are "built to play and built by play." He encourages health and wellness practitioners to "prescribe free play." You can learn more at **nifplay.org**.

A Course in Miracles (ACIM) is a spiritual self-study program designed to awaken us to the truth of love and our Oneness with all of life. Psychologist Helen Schucman scribed it through a process of inner dictation. The entire text of ACIM, its workbook, and its teaching manual are available for free at **acim.org**.

Corinne Cayce is an integral life coach and the great-granddaughter of Edgar Cayce, the renowned American psychic. Her work inspired part of the dream analysis section in this book. Corinne and I also cohost the parenting podcast ***Edgar Cayce's Creating Calm: Parenting with Mind, Body, and Spirit*** which can be found on most podcasting platforms. Corinne's website is **caycecoaching.com**.

Edgar Cayce's Association for Research and Enlightenment (A.R.E.) is a nonprofit dedicated to preserving his work. Cayce is the most well-studied psychic of the twentieth century. He gave over 14,000 recorded psychic readings, most of which were on health and healing, including recommendations on the **alkaline diet**. The Cayce readings also emphasized that we are each a part of the Love and Oneness. You can learn more at **edgarcayce.org**.

The ***Edgar Cayce Readings Dream Dictionary*** lists symbols clearly interpreted in one or more of Edgar Cayce's readings on dreams. You can use these as a starting point, keeping in mind that dreams are personal and symbols carry many interpretations. This dream dictionary

is available online or as an app. Go to **edgarcayce.org/the-readings/
dreams/dream-dictionary/**.

Gary Craig founded the **Emotional Freedom Technique (EFT)** in
1995. EFT involves tapping on acupressure points to relieve energetic
blockages and restore physical and emotional balance. Gary's newest
work involves a more spiritual approach called **Optimal EFT**. You can
learn more about both versions of EFT at **emofree.com**.

Deborah Craydon is a certified flower essence practitioner and creator of **Flora Corona**, a company that focuses on vibrational elixirs,
including gem, color, and Hawaiian flower essences, as well as online
trainings. She and acupuncturist Warren Bellows coauthored the book
*Floral Acupuncture: Applying the Flower Essences of Dr. Bach to
Acupuncture Sites.* Learn more at **floracorona.com**.

Masaru Emoto was a businessman who studied water for over twenty
years. He found that water has memory and is connected to our
individual and collective consciousness. Loving thoughts influence
water molecules to form beautiful snowflake patterns while unloving
thoughts result in disorganized molecular patterns. You can see photographs of this in Emoto's *New York Times* bestselling book, *The Hidden
Messages in Water*. You can also learn more at **masaru-emoto.net**.

The HeartMath Institute, founded by Doc Childre, has conducted
groundbreaking research on the human heart field and consciousness.
HeartMath's vision is to provide people with tools to connect us with
"the heart of who we truly are." They provide biofeedback programs
and meditations to help improve heart coherence for overall health
and well-being. Learn more at **heartmath.com**.

Ingrid Fetell is a designer and author whose popular **TED talk**
"Where Joy Hides and How to Find It" has had millions of views. She
talks about the influence color and shapes have on our emotions and
well-being. She is also the author of *Joyful: The Surprising Power of
Ordinary Things to Create Extraordinary Happiness.* You can learn
more at **aestheticsofjoy.com**.

Maudy Fowler is a spiritual consultant and author of many books, including *Angel Whispers* and *Angel Messages.* She has the gift of clear-hearing, or clairaudience. You can join one of her inspirational groups by emailing her at **maudyandgail@aol.com** or through her website, **maudy.com**.

Charlie Goldsmith is an energy healer whose healing abilities have been studied jointly by Monash University Professor Paul Komeseroff (in Australia) and the NYU Lutheran Hospital in New York City. His work was featured in the TLC television series *The Healer.* You can learn more at **charliegoldsmith.com**.

Louise Hay was an author and speaker whose emphasis on positive affirmations helped spark the self-help movement. She founded the publishing company Hay House, Inc. Her book *You Can Heal Your Life* is a New York Times bestseller with more than 50 million copies sold worldwide. Learn more at **louisehay.com**.

Shawn Marie Higgins, DO, is an osteopathic physician and sound healer who teaches courses on vibrational and sound healing globally. She explains the relationship between sound, quantum physics, and consciousness. You can learn more about Dr. Higgins at **osteopathicwell.com**.

Shamini Jain, PhD, is a psychologist and researcher whose ground-breaking book *Healing Ourselves: Biofield Science and the Future of Health* received the 2022 Nautilus Award. She founded the **Consciousness and Healing Initiative** (CHI), "a nonprofit collaborative of scientists, practitioners, educators, innovators, and artists dedicated to leading humanity to heal ourselves." Learn more about Dr. Jain at **shaminijain.com** and CHI at **chi.is**.

Melissa Joy Jonsson is an author, speaker, and creator of the Joy Mapping process. She is Dr. Richard Bartlett's longtime co-teacher and has been teaching popular life-transforming seminars worldwide since 2008. With a background in neuroscience, psychology, and intuitive healing, she teaches people the science of heart-centered awareness. Learn more at **melissajoy.com.**

Anne Lamott is an author and speaker who tells stories with raw honesty and compassion. Her *New York Times* bestselling book *Bird by Bird: Some Instructions on Writing and Life* has inspired countless writers and creatives. She has been inducted into the California Hall of Fame.

Michael Lennox is a psychologist, renowned dream expert, and author of *Dream Sight: A Dictionary and Guide for Interpreting Any Dream.* He also runs a Dream Circle. You can learn more at **michaellennox.com.**

Jacob Liberman, OD, PhD, is an optometrist and vision scientist investigating the relationship between light, vision, and consciousness for over forty years. He has invented multiple phototherapy systems to improve visual performance. You can learn more from his book *Luminous Life: How the Science of Light Unlocks the Art of Living* and his website at **jacobliberman.org.**

Bruce Lipton, PhD, is a stem cell biologist and bestselling author of *The Biology of Belief: Unleashing the Power of Consciousness, Matter, and Miracles.* His breakthrough research has helped us better understand how quantum physics applies to our cells and how consciousness influences the expression of our genes. He received the 2009 Goi Peace Award for his work. Learn more at **brucelipton.com.**

Tieraoni Low Dog, MD, is a physician, herbalist, author, and speaker in integrative medicine. She was the former Fellowship Director at the University of Arizona Center for Integrative Medicine, has chaired dietary supplement expert panels for the United States Pharmacopeia, and has served on numerous advisory panels. Dr. Low Dog has authored many bestselling books, including *Life is Your Best Medicine.* Learn more at **drlowdog.com.**

Gladys McGarey, MD, physician and cofounder of the American Holistic Medical Association, has helped transform how we look at health and self-care. She is often referred to as the mother of holistic medicine. A centenarian, she is the author of *The Well-Lived Life: A 102-Year-Old Doctor's Six Secrets to Health and Happiness at Every Age.* You can learn more about her at **gladysmcgarey.com**.

Lynne McTaggart is an award-winning journalist and author of multiple books, including the international bestsellers *The Power of Eight, The Field, The Intention Experiment,* and *The Bond.* Her work focuses on the power of intention and consciousness. You can learn more about Lynne and her ongoing group intention experiments at **lynnemctaggart.com**.

Pamela Miles is the foremost medical Reiki expert. Collaborating with major medical institutions, including the National Institutes of Health (NIH), Harvard, Yale, Einstein, and other major medical centers, she pioneered the use of Reiki in conventional medicine. She is also the author of *Reiki: A Comprehensive Guide.* Learn more at **pamelamiles. com** and **reikiinmedicine.com**.

Anita Moorjani is a speaker and author of multiple books, including the New York Times bestseller *Dying to Be Me: My Journey from Cancer, to Near Death, to True Healing,* which details her near-death experience with clarity. She also wrote *Sensitive is the New Strong: The Power of Empaths in an Increasingly Harsh World.* You can learn more at **anitamoorjani.com**.

Peter Reynolds is a writer, storyteller, and illustrator whose inspirational books have received numerous awards. His book *The Dot* has been published in over twenty languages, including Braille. His bookstore, The Blue Bunny Books and Toys, is located just outside Boston. To access his online shop, go to **thedotcentral.com**. To learn more about Peter, go to **peterhreynolds.com**.

Shunryu Suzuki was a Sōtō Zen monk who founded the San Francisco Zen Center. His book *Zen Mind, Beginner's Mind: Informal Talks on Zen Meditation and Practice* has become a modern Zen classic. Emmy award-winning actor Peter Coyote narrates the audio version of the book.

SpiritQuest Sedona Retreats offers **customized retreats** to enhance **personal growth and healing.** I've sent many people there to help remind themselves of who they already are. As it says on their website, "There's only one soul in all of creation you can truly know, and it's the one whose fate is placed in your hands." ~C.S. Lewis. You can learn more at **retreatsinsedona.com.**

Jill Sylvester is a licensed mental health counselor, speaker, host of the *Trust Your Intuition* **podcast,** and author of the young adult novel *The Land of Blue,* a Mom's Choice Award winner; *Trust Your Intuition: 100 Ways to Transform Anxiety and Depression for Stronger Mental Health,* a Nautilus Award winner; and the young *adult* **Devon: Dream Agent** series exploring empathic abilities and mental-emotional health. Learn more at **jillsylvester.com.**

Mai Trinh, MS, CHHC, is the founder of **Mai Health Now** and author of **The Glee Method.** Focusing on **Chronic Disease Prevention,** she is a sought-after speaker for Fortune 500 companies, federal and local government agencies, and other organizations. Mai also works with individual clients on mindset, energy, sleep, nutrition, and overall happiness. Learn more at **maihealthnow.com.**

Neale Donald Walsch is a spiritual messenger and author of the *Conversations with God* book series. I noted his definition of hope in the last book of the series, *Home with God*: "Hope is thought made Divine." You can learn more at **nealedonaldwalsch.com.**

Andrew Weil, MD, is a global leader and pioneer in integrative medicine. He is the founder and director of the Andrew Weil Center for Integrative Medicine at the University of Arizona and the author of many books, including the *New York Times* bestseller *Spontaneous Healing.* He and Dr. Victoria Maizes cohost the podcast *Body of Wonder.* You can learn more about integrative medicine at **drweil.com** and his fellowship for healthcare practitioners at **integrativemedicine.arizona.edu**.

NOTES

Chapter 1: A New Way of Looking at Symptoms

1. In this book, sometimes I use the terms "layers" and "dimensions" interchangeably when referring to the physical, mental, emotional, and spiritual aspects of our being. By "layers," I do not mean layers like an onion. Rather, they are interpenetrating dimensions of our being. These dimensions are also part of our subtle energy body, or biofield. More on our subtle energy body later in Chapter 1.

2. The "incoordination of the nervous system" is a phrase Edgar Cayce often used. The most well-documented medical psychic of the twentieth century, Edgar was a huge proponent of holistic health.

3. Lauri Nummenmaa, Enrico Glerean, et al., "Bodily maps of emotions," *Proceedings of the National Academy of Sciences* 111, no. 2 (December 2013): 646–651.

4. The concept of the body and brain functioning on half-battery was introduced to me by my good friend and colleague Maria Coffman, DO, and is based on Donna Eden's work on the body's various energy systems.

5. Carla Hannaford, *Smart Moves: Why Learning Is Not All in Your Head* (Salt Lake City: Great River Books, 2005).

Chapter 2: Grounding the Body and Opening the Heart

1. The Environmental Working Group is a 30-million-strong community working to protect our environmental health by changing industry standards; learn more at ewg.org.

2. Ibid.

3. The Dirty Dozen™ is the Environmental Working Group's

shopper's guide to pesticides in products; see ewg.org/food-news/dirty-dozen.php.

4. Most healthy diets are variations of the alkaline diet which focuses on whole, preservative-free, alkaline-forming foods with more leafy greens than starchy vegetables. The Mediterranean diet is an example of an alkaline diet. For a downloadable handout on the alkaline diet, go to allworldspress.com.

5. James L Oschman, Gaétan Chevalier, and Richard Brown, "The Effects of Grounding (Earthing) on Inflammation, the Immune Response, Wound Healing, and Prevention and Treatment of Chronic Inflammatory and Autoimmune Diseases," *Journal of Inflammation Research* 8 (March 2015): 83–96.

6. Wendy Menigoz, Tracy Latz, Robin Ely, Cimone Kamei, Gregory Melvin, and Drew Sinatra. "Integrative and lifestyle medicine strategies should include Earthing (grounding): Review of research evidence and clinical observations," *Explore* 16, no. 3 (May-June 2020) 152-160.

7. Rikuto Yamashita, Chong Chen, et al., "The Mood-Improving Effect of Viewing Images of Nature and Its Neural Substrate," *The International Journal of Environmental Research and Public Health* 18, no. 10 (May 2021): 5500.

8. "Epigenetic Control of Gene Expression," a Coursera class taught by Dr. Marnie Blewitt, Head of the Molecular Medicine Laboratory at the University of Melbourne; see coursera.org/learn/epigenetics.

9. Bruce Lipton, *The Biology of Belief: 10th Anniversary Edition* (Carlsbad, CA: Hay House, 2016).

Part 1: Exercises for the Intuitive Body

1. Jonathan Goldman and Andi Goldman, *The Humming Effect: Sound Healing for Health and Happiness* (Rochester, Vermont: Healing Arts, 2017).

2. This is a variation on a meditation inspired by Deborah Craydon, a flower essence practitioner and author of *Floral Acupuncture: Applying the Flower Essences of Dr. Bach to Acupuncture Sites* (Crossing Press, 2005).

Chapter 4: Thoughts—What Are They?

1. "The Power of the Placebo Effect," Harvard Health Publishing, December23,2021;health.harvard.edu/mental-health/the-power-of-the-placebo-effect.

2. Saul McLeod, "Cognitive Approach in Psychology," simplypsychology.org.

3. S. K. Pandya, "Understanding Brain, Mind and Soul: Contributions from Neurology and Neurosurgery," *Mens Sana Monographs* 9, no. 1 (2011): 129–149.

4. E. S. Krishnamoorthy, "When Your Mind and Soul Meet," *The Hindu Magazine*, August 31, 2009.

5. Karen Rommelfanger, PhD, is Program Director of the Neuroethics Program at the Ethics Center, associate professor in the Departments of Neurology and Psychiatry at Emory University, and scientific collaborator for Terminus Modern Ballet Theatre. Panel discussion at end of performance on May 18, 2021, hosted by Georgia Tech Arts.

6. There are many definitions for the terms outlined in the table "Working Definitions of Mind, Thought, and Consciousness." My definition of "consciousness" corresponds with Edgar Cayce's term "universal consciousness," or "higher consciousness," or "super consciousness." Although the subconscious is under ordinary awareness, it is also so much more. With practice, the subconscious can become a channel of higher consciousness and receive continuous guidance from the universal Oneness.

7. See the "Recommended Resources" in this book for more information on Richard Bartlett, Melissa Joy, and Matrix Energetics.

8. Shunryu Suzuki, *Zen Mind, Beginner's Mind: 50th Anniversary Edition* (Boulder, Colorado: Shambhala, 2020).

9. "Human Body May Be 99% Water Reports Water Researcher Gerald Pollack, PhD," prweb.com, February 27, 2014.

10. Masaru Emoto, *The Hidden Messages in Water* (New York: Atria Books, 2005).

11. This method was inspired by the late Marcel Vogel and his

crystal healing techniques. Vogel was a research scientist who worked with IBM for 27 years. He had many inventions including the Liquid Crystalline Display (LCD). As Vogel explained, when we inhale our intention and hold our breath, a charge carrying the message is built up in your energy body. Then, as we exhale, the message is released around us. The use of a quick and directed outbreath through the nostrils helps to consolidate the message so that it is directed into the water or crystal with laser-like action. Here is one video with Marcel Vogel discussing the therapeutic use of crystals: www.youtube.com/watch?v=6c9HQ4lM8JY.

Chapter 5: Grounding the Mind

1. Carl Jung, *Modern Man in Search of a Soul* (Eastford, Connecticut: Martino Fine Books, 2017), p. 242. (*Modern Man in Search of a Soul* was first published in 1933.)

2. Emily Alfin Johnson and Lisa Weiner, "App Lets You Destress By Screaming Into Icelandic Wilderness," npr.org, July 17, 2020.

3. Anne Lamott, *Almost Everything: Notes on Hope* (New York: Riverhead Books, 2018).

Chapter 8: Grounding the Spirit

1. *A Course in Miracles,* Text, Chapter 3, Part V (Novato, California: Foundation for Inner Peace, 1975).

2. Archbishop Desmond Tutu, "Ubuntu: The Essence of Being Human," YouTube.com; youtube.com/watch?v=44xbZ8M-N1uk; accessed December 17, 2023.

Chapter 9: Your Spirit As Your Compass

1. Jacob Liberman, *Luminous Life: How the Science of Light Unlocks the Art of Living* (Novato, California: New World Library, 2018).

2. Tai chi and other martial arts emphasize a relaxed strength that is stronger than a tense strength.

3. The dream tips come from Corinne Cayce and Arlene Dijamco.

Chapter 10: The Art of Intuitive Living

1. "What Is Play?" National Institute for Play; nifplay.org/what-is-play/the-basics/.

2. "What Are Your Play Personalities?" National Institute for Play; nifplay.org/what-is-play/play-personalities/.

Chapter 11: Multidimensional Medicine

1. Colin P. West, Angelina D. Tan, et al., "Association of Resident Fatigue and Distress with Perceived Medical Errors," *Journal of American Medical Association* 302, no. 12 (September 2009): 1294–1300.

2. Jill Suttie, "How Kindness Fits into a Happy Life," Greater Good Magazine, greatergood.berkeley.edu, February 17, 2021.

3. "The Science of Kindness," Cedars-Sinai Blog, cedars-sinai.org/blog/science-of-kindness.html, February 13, 2019.

4. Greater Good Magazine, https://greatergood.berkeley.edu/.

5. Louise B. Andrew, Barry E. Breener, et al., "Physician Suicide," Medscape, July 13, 2022; https://emedicine.medscape.com/article/806779-overview?form=fpf.

6. Tait D. Shanafelt, Colin P. West, et al., "Changes in Burnout and Satisfaction With Work-Life Integration in Physicians Over the First 2 Years of the COVID-19 Pandemic," *Mayo Clinic Proceedings* 97, no. 12 (December 2022): 2248–2258; mayoclinicproceedings.org/article/S0025-6196(22)00515-8/fulltext.

7. Claire Parker, "U.S. Healthcare System Ranks Last Among 11 High-Income Countries, Researchers Say," washingtonpost.com, August 5, 2021.

8. Linda Carroll, "Prescriptions for Healthy Food Might Save Lives—and Money," reuters.com, March 19, 2019; also see Yujin Lee, Dariush Mozaffarian, et al., "Cost-effectiveness of Financial Incentives for Improving Diet and Health through Medicare and Medicaid: A Microsimulation Study," *PLOS Medicine* 16, no. 3 (March 2019): e1002761.

INDEX OF EXERCISES

ACKNOWLEDGMENTS

I would like to extend my heartfelt thanks for the many friends, family, and loved ones who supported me in the creation of this book. You are all a part of my soul family. I am filled with warm, fuzzy feelings of love when I think of each of you.

First off, my parents, who paved the way for me with their endless dedication, from answering the phone at all hours, to impromptu feasts "just because," to rushing a computer to me when mine crashed. You are my earth angels. And Dad, now you are one of my pure spirit angels as well. Your guidance from spirit has been more than I could have imagined. I could not have written this book without the constant dialogue we share.

To my husband Greg, who has believed in me always and has lifted me up through all the behind-the-scenes work that it takes to put together yet another monumental project. Thank you for all that you are and do. There are not enough words. *I am because you are.*

To my kids, who have seen their mommy through thick and thin and cheered me on, adding their pearls of wisdom along the way. You are all old souls, and I cherish your love.

To my siblings, you have enriched me with fun explorations through all the weather life brings. Your curiosity, laughter, honesty, and enduring love are constant reminders of what family is all about. To my cousins, aunts, uncles, and all the Titas and Titos I thought were related to me, too—thanks for setting the backdrop of a nurturing extended family. To my cousin Ryan in particular, who shared in detail his NDE and spiritual journey and who heard the message loud and clear that *everybody is waking up*, delivered in a humorous Peppa Pig voice (stories for another book!)

To my Lola, who has been a guiding angel throughout my medical education and beyond. She taught me about the beauty in colors, patterns, and foods, and how when you don't know how big to make something, just measure it! *Collect your data points.*

To my in-laws, Jim and Sharon, and all the Botelho family, thanks for listening to my stories for many years now and for sharing them with friends and neighbors.

To my childhood friends Betsey, Carrie, Emily, Minesh, and Sheva, we have each other's backs no matter what. As they say, *good friends are like stars—you don't always see them, but you know they're always there.*

To my physician friends and colleagues, including many insightful conversations with James Gaydos, DO, my co-teacher for the Dig On Series—Exploring Consciousness Through Osteopathy; Shawn Marie Higgins, DO sound healer and author who inspired the conversation on the Fibonacci sequence; Maria Coffman, DO author of *Booby Traps: A Book of Bras, Breasts, and Bands*; and Lilia Gorodinsky, DO, of nyosteo.com. You are all osteopathic physicians extraordinaire. Thank you for encouraging me to speak.

To my healer friends who have kept me company over the years: Maudy Fowler, a spiritual consultant and bestselling author of *Angel Messages*; Pamela Miles, the world's foremost medical Reiki expert; Maxine Taylor, the first licensed astrologist in the US; Sheri Baker, a spiritual teacher of *A Course in Miracles* and Optimal EFT; and Deborah Craydon, a pioneer in floral acupuncture. I treasure your ongoing love and support.

To Corinne Cayce, an integral life coach and great-granddaughter of Edgar Cayce, you are a true soul sister. I'm so thankful to co-host the parenting podcast *Edgar Cayce's Creating Calm* with you, and I look forward to many more adventures together.

To the many people whose work and stories I've shared in this book, including those mentioned in the reference section. To Marianne Ellis, who shared her practice of intuitive photography and art (find her work on instagram.com/soul_reflectioncoach/). To Travis Carr, who shares his love of art and people so freely. To Brian Sutton, my tai chi instructor, who helped me improve my balance, flexibility, and strength. To Suzanne Lye, a professor of classics who gives life to the word *humanity* and the study of the humanities.

To my many patients, I have learned so much from all of you over the years. This book is for you. You asked for it, and here it is! You are all a big part of what gives this book so much heart.

To Dacey Paul, you are more than an office manager, more than a naturopath, more than a life essence coach—you are my friend. Thank you for aligning your heart, mind, and spirit with the overarching vision of the All Worlds Family, the Dig On Series, and now the School of Stillness.

To Mai Trinh, my book-writing partner and dear friend, who has met with me and our book coach every two weeks for the last two years! My, how we've grown! You are an amazing holistic health counselor with your own book, *The Glee Method*.

To all my beta-readers: Steve Wan, Kelli Haxel, Susie and Graciela Lotharius, Maria Coffman, Sue Radics, Courtney Peters, and Starlight Katsaros, thank you all for your insightful feedback, encouragement, and ongoing support of me, the book, and the purpose: *to know yourself and express the love that you are.* I am growing and celebrating with you.

To my book team, including Michelle Bish, the best book coach ever; Vesela Simic, the editor of my dreams; Diane Rigoli, my book designer, who made it visually beautiful; Caitlin Tabilog, who makes photoshoots fun; and Jennifer Hamady, my voice coach, who helped me prep for the audiobook recording. Writing, recording, and publishing a book is like having a baby, and I feel like a new mom again! Thanks for making the process so much easier.

To my readers, through you this book lives on. I believe in you, and I hope you believe in you, too.

To all of you, I am forever grateful.

With love,

Arlene

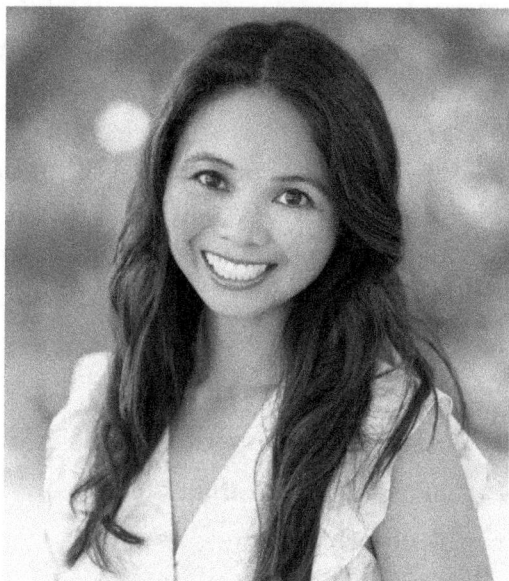

ABOUT THE AUTHOR

DR. ARLENE DIJAMCO, THE MULTIDIMENSIONAL MD, is an integrative physician, pediatrician, and cranial osteopath who is passionate about making the intangible aspects of health—the energetic, mental, emotional, and spiritual—more practical for people. She studied at Harvard University, Emory University, and the Albert Einstein College of Medicine, but her therapeutic toolbox expanded tremendously after completing Dr. Andrew Weil's two-year integrative medicine fellowship at the University of Arizona. Dr. Dijamco is known for her intuitive knack and her abilities to connect with and empower people to nourish and balance all dimensions of their health. She serves on the faculty of the Osteopathic Cranial Academy and with Edgar Cayce's Association for Research and Enlightenment; she also teaches Tension and Trauma Release Exercises around the country. She founded and oversees All Worlds Health, which includes her medical practice near Atlanta, Georgia, as well as a nonprofit and a publishing company. Dr. Dijamco recently launched two teaching programs: The

Dig On Series—Exploring Consciousness Through Osteopathy, for osteopaths, and School of Stillness—Where Everyone Is a Healer, for wellness practitioners and all explorers interested in self-development. She also hosts two podcasts: *The MultiDimensional MD* on YouTube and *Edgar Cayce's Creating Calm—Parenting with Mind, Body, and Spirit*, with co-host Corinne Cayce, which can be found on most podcasting platforms including Spotify and Apple. *Atlanta Modern & Luxury* named her a leader in wellness. At home, she is a yoga novice, an awesome wife, and mom to four incredible girls. Learn more about Dr. Dijamco at allworldshealth.com.

- Publishing website: **allworldspress.com**
- Practice website: **allworldshealth.com**
- The Dig On Series: **thedigonseries.com**
- School of Stillness: **schoolofstillness.org**
- Instagram: **@allworldshealth**
- Facebook: **/allworldshealthandpediatrics**
- *Edgar Cayce's Creating Calm—Parenting with Mind, Body, and Spirit* podcast: **edgarcayce.org/groups-services/family-resource-hub/listen/** and other podcasting platforms.
- *The MultiDimensional MD* podcast on YouTube: **youtube.com/c/arlenedijamcomd** and other podcasting platforms.

www.ingramcontent.com/pod-product-compliance
Lightning Source LLC
Chambersburg PA
CBHW031546260326
41914CB00002B/286

* 9 7 8 1 9 6 3 8 9 9 0 0 9 *